About The Author

D1784961

Many years ago, I was diagnosed with an incurable disease. It's an unknown autoimmune disease that left me bedridden occasionally and immobile frequently for some time. According to the doctor, the cause is unknown. I was devastated. I used to be athletic. All of a sudden, I couldn't even walk properly, let alone going for sports activities.

Desperate for healing, I went to chiropractors, orthopedics, rheumatologists and many other doctors, but to no avail. None of them could do anything to help relieve my symptoms (excruciating pain all over my body) except to deplete most of my savings.

It was then that I turned to a Supreme Being for help. Soon, I discovered **the Secret to Divine Healing**. After some time, my symptoms began to fade off. Eventually, every symptom and pain in my body left! I stopped taking all the medication ---- mostly painkillers and steroids. Being convinced that I was healed, I went back to the doctor for a medical review. The medical report showed that my blood was the same as that of an average person, and there was no more inflammation in my body! The doctor was amazed, and exclaimed, *"What did you do to your body?"*

It has been 7 years since I received my healing, and today, I stand healed, healthy and strong. I have regained my exercise regime and I am living my life with a burning passion to see others healed completely ------- regardless of their sickness or disease. I have seen thousands of individuals healed everywhere I go as a lifestyle, and I am talking about individuals ------ one person at a time in the streets. This does not include groups and multitudes in healing meetings and services.

What I am going to share with you in this manual is **simple**. Having said that, it is important to know that while the distance between the head and the heart is only 18 inches, yet for some people, the journey from head to the heart can take several years. I have seen people who received this simple truth on divine healing and received their healing immediately.

One example is a lady who had a lump in her breast disappearing immediately after hearing this simple truth. Another was healed from childhood epilepsy when she went back for a brain scan. Nobody ministered healing to them! There were many more, of which I could not possibly list them all in this manual.

This manual contains mostly teachings, instead of stories. Stories inspire and encourage you, but only teachings will impart truths into your life that will set you free and keep you free. I have scores of testimonies to share, but that is not as vital as the teachings. If you get the foundation right, you will have your own testimonies.

I would like to request that you do not rush through reading this manual. **DO NOT SKIP** through the pages. Take time to slowly digest the words from each chapter. Each page lays foundation upon foundation so that you can truly **BELIEVE**. I believe that divine healing is **YOURS**!

© Copyright Y.Z. Wilson Barnabas, 2019

All rights reserved under International Copyright Law.

Published by:

INDEPENDENT PUBLISHER

Unless otherwise stated, all quotations from Scriptures are taken from the New King James Version.

Contents may not be reproduced in whole or in part in any form without the express written consent of the author.

Printed in the United States of America

Content

Chapter 1:
The Great Redemption

I have researched and studied a lot about healing for many years. I listened to all kinds of video and audio messages about healing. I also go out to minister healing to others. I am determined to see divine healing taking place in the lives of people.

Today, there are many messages on divine healing out there, but many of them are not Scripture-based. Some of them interpret the Scriptures based on their experiences. That is deductive, rather than inductive. What I am sharing in this manual can be tested by the Scriptures. Don't just take everything wholesale. Be like the Bereans. Search the Scriptures on this manual. It is worth your time to read and meditate on the Word on your own, so that you can establish the truths within your heart and not be wavered by every kind of doctrine.

Divine Healing is SIMPLE! Therefore, everything I am going to share will be simple. It simply takes a believing heart to receive this.

God Did Not Create Man To Have Sickness Or Death

In the very beginning, God created Man to live forever on earth because Man was created in God's image (Genesis 1:26-27).

*And the Lord God commanded the man, saying, "Of every tree of the garden you may freely eat; but of the **tree of the knowledge of good and evil** you shall not eat, for in the day that you eat of it **you shall surely die**.* - Genesis 2:16-17

If Adam did not eat the fruit from the tree of the knowledge of good and evil, he would have enjoyed eternal life with His Creator by partaking the tree of life.

*"...And now, lest he put out his hand and take also of the **tree of life**, and eat, and **live forever**"— therefore the Lord God sent him out of*

3

the garden of Eden to till the ground from which he was taken. So He drove out the man; and He placed cherubim at the east of the garden of Eden, and a flaming sword which turned every way, to guard the way to the tree of life. - Genesis 3:22-24

God, in His wisdom and love, had to guard the tree of life from Adam, so that he would not **live in sin** FOREVER.

Despite his Fall, Adam died at the age of 930 (Genesis 5:5). Today, we think that we can only live till 80 because experience and the medical world have become our teachers. **The Word of God should be our teacher!**

Because of sin, death entered the world (Romans 5:12). The First Adam's offense resulted in sickness and death in all mankind. But the Good News is this ----- Jesus, the Last Adam came to remove sin from us, so that **we can be redeemed from sickness and death!**

*"Behold! The Lamb of God who **takes away** the sin of the world!"* - John 1:29

He has appeared to **put away sin** by the sacrifice of Himself. - Hebrews 9:26

*For if by the one man's offense death reigned through the one, much more those who receive abundance of grace and of the gift of righteousness will **reign in life through the One, Jesus Christ**.* - Romans 5:17

Since Jesus was the One who redeemed us from sin, we must look at His life and His finished works on the Cross. This is the **KEY** to receive divine healing!

Jesus Is The Exact Representation Of God

This is a simple truth, but many people overlook it. If we want to know how God looks like in nature and character, we can simply look at Jesus in the four books of the Gospel. Jesus is God manifested in the flesh (John 1:1; 1 John 1:1-2).

*The Son is the radiance of God's glory and the **exact representation** of His being.* - Hebrews 1:3

*No one has ever seen God; the only Son, who is at the Father's side, **He has made Him known**.* - John 1:18

In other words, everything that Jesus said and did throughout the books of the Gospel is exactly what God the Father wanted to say and do (John 5:19). Jesus revealed the perfect will of God!

When Jesus *spoke*, it was the Father who *wanted* to speak.
When Jesus *healed*, it was the Father who *wanted* to heal.

More than 30% of the books of the Gospel are all on healing. And almost 50% of Jesus' ministry recorded in the Gospel is on healing. This means that healing is an integral part of the Gospel. You cannot know Jesus more without knowing His heart for healing.

When Jesus healed the leper, He said, "*I am willing, be cleansed.*" (Matthew 8:3) The word 'willing' is not a good English translation. It does not simply mean that Jesus is willing to make him clean. The word 'willing' in the Greek means 'to will, to desire, to have in mind.' It speaks of the **nature of God, who He is**. He is Jehovah Rapha, the Lord our Healer (Exodus 15:26). The nature of God refers to His will - "*It is who I AM.*"

So when Jesus healed, He didn't heal merely because He was willing. He healed because **it was His nature and His will to heal**. In fact, everyone who came to Him was healed.

*How God anointed Jesus of Nazareth with the Holy Spirit and with power, who went about doing good and **healing all** who were **oppressed by the devil**, for God was with Him.* - Acts 10:38

Jesus did not heal some. He healed ALL. He wasn't picking and choosing who He should heal. He healed ALL, regardless of their sicknesses, diseases, situations, and backgrounds. Notice, the verse says '*healing all who were oppressed by the devil*.' Herein lies the clear revelation of where the root of sickness came from ------- the devil. When you learn how to deal with sickness the same way you would deal with the enemy, you will experience healing! We will talk more about this in the later part of this manual.

Jesus Is The Perfect Interpretation Of Who God Is

When you do not understand the nature of God in your situation, always go back and look at Jesus in the Word and what He has done on the Cross. Never second-guess how God looks like based on your own experience, and others' interpretations. Even the preachers at the pulpit may present God wrongly to you. Therefore, it is important to be like the Bereans, whom the Bible said were of noble character because they examined the Scriptures (Acts 17:11) and didn't follow the pulpit's teachings blindly.

God does NOT punish or judge you with sickness. Neither does He allow sickness so that you can learn something, whether its patience or growth in character. You can't find a single record where Jesus judged someone with sickness or tolerated sickness so that someone could grow in character. He always healed and delivered them all (Matthew 8:16).

*And Jesus went about all Galilee, teaching in their synagogues, preaching the gospel of the kingdom, and **healing <u>all</u> kinds of sickness** and **<u>all</u> kinds of disease** among the people.* - Matthew 4:23

Each time when you have a thought about God that is not consistent with what you see in Jesus, that is NOT God.

*The thief comes only to steal and kill and destroy; **I came that they may have life**, and have it abundantly.* - John 10:10

Jesus' words are very simple. But we tend to make them complicated. Life comes from Him. Anything that does not give life is not from Him. When bad things come into your life; when sickness comes, it is not God who gives it to you. **It is the enemy. He has come to steal, kill and destroy.**

In the context of this passage, Jesus was talking about the false teachers, who came from the father of lies (John 8:44). When you listen to lies (i.e. maybe God doesn't want to heal me yet) and accept them, you give room for the enemy to steal, kill and destroy. **Remember: Half-truths are still lies!** If you believe that God is the One causing the sickness, you won't be able to receive healing. If you believe that it is not God's timing to heal you NOW, you won't be able to receive healing.

Jesus Is The Same Yesterday, Today And Forever

Because Jesus never changes (Hebrews 13:8), whatever He does and says is eternal and permanent. **He doesn't change His mind on healing you.** He doesn't change His mind on delivering you. He doesn't change His mind in giving you life!

Some of you may wonder, "Why does God seem to be different in the Old Testament? Didn't He judge the people with afflictions?"

We must understand what happened on the Cross that changed everything!

Jesus' Perfect Sacrifice on the Cross

Before Christ came, we were living under the law of sin and death (Romans 8:2). Under the Law, if you walk in obedience, a list of blessings would come upon you (Deuteronomy 28:1-14). On the other hand, if you walk in disobedience or sin, a list of curses would come upon you (Deuteronomy 28:15-68). This was the reason why people were judged in the Old Covenant when they sinned.

No one in history had ever fulfilled all the requirements of the Law, except for Jesus while He was on earth. God sent His only begotten Son to redeem us from this curse of the Law (Galatians 3:13). Why did God do so?

God is Love, but He is also a Righteous Judge. To love effectively, one has to judge effectively. God loves us deeply. As such, He had to judge sin, because sin would destroy us (Romans 6:23; James 1:15).

The effects of sin are sicknesses, broken relationships, death, etc. God wanted to set mankind free from this cycle of sin and death. The only way was to send His Son to fulfill all the requirements of the Law, walked blamelessly, lived without sin and offered Himself as the perfect sacrifice to redeem us from judgment and sin!

*Therefore, as through one man's offense judgment came to all men, resulting in condemnation, even so through one Man's righteous act the free gift came to all men, **resulting in justification of life**.* - Romans 5:18

*All have sinned and fall short of the glory of God, being justified freely by His grace through the **redemption that is in Christ Jesus**, whom God set forth as a propitiation by His blood, through faith, to demonstrate His righteousness, because in His forbearance **God had passed over the sins that were previously committed**, to demonstrate at the present time His righteousness, that **He might be just and the justifier of the one who has faith in Jesus**.* - Romans 3:23-36

In sending Jesus to redeem us, God demonstrated His righteousness and justice to forgive every sin that He didn't judge from the Old Testament to our days. Jesus is God's righteousness revealed (Romans 1:16-17). This is why He could go around forgiving the sins of people (Matthew 9:6; Mark 2:5; Luke 7:48; John 8:11) in the books of the Gospel because He would eventually pay for them on the Cross.

Jesus Himself came on earth to fulfill the Law (Matthew 5:17-18). Since the age of 12 (Luke 2:42), Jesus obeyed every requirement of the Law. According to the Jewish custom, you become an adult at the age of 12 and your responsibility to keep the Law begins. After Jesus was baptized in the water, the Bible (Matthew 3:15) says that He fulfilled all righteousness (all requirements of the Law). Because of the fulfillment of the Law, all the blessings in Deuteronomy 28 came upon Jesus ------ the Spirit of God descended upon Jesus (Matthew 3:16). Heaven was opened for Jesus!

Something similar happened on the Cross. Jesus had to be hung on the Cross in order to become a curse. Without dying on the Cross, He would not be able to free us from the curse of the Law.

*Christ has **redeemed us from the curse of the law**, having become a curse for us (for it is written, "Cursed is everyone who hangs on a tree").* - Galatians 3:13

When Jesus was hung on the Cross, He took upon our sin and became the curse (2 Corinthians 5:21) so that we might become the righteousness of God in Him. **God destroyed the curse of sin in the body of His Son, so that we can be free from the penalty and effects of sin once and for all!**

By doing that, we are made right with God. God now sees us as if we have fulfilled all the righteous requirement of the Law!

When Jesus fulfilled all righteousness after He was baptized in water, heaven was opened for Him (Mark 1:10). When Jesus died on the Cross and fulfilled all righteousness **in us**, heaven is opened for us (Matthew 27:51).

*He condemned sin in the flesh, in order that the **righteous requirement of the law might be fulfilled in us**, who walk not according to the flesh but according to the Spirit.* - Romans 8:3-4

As believers, heaven is permanently opened for us, and there is nothing we can do to shut heaven's door because it wasn't open by your efforts or works. It was opened by the finished works of Jesus on the Cross! This gives us access to every spiritual blessing (Ephesians 1:3) including HEALING!

We Are Now In Christ (The New Covenant)

A covenant requires two parties. A benefactor and a beneficiary. God is usually the benefactor and man is the beneficiary. A covenant is more than a contract. It binds a relationship together. There are different covenants in the Bible, but for the purpose of divine healing, we will look at the covenant that we are in.

The Old Covenant is the law of sin and death, where the beneficiary receives either blessings or curses depending on his act of obedience.

The New Covenant is the law of the Spirit (Romans 8:2), where we become the beneficiaries because we are IN Christ.

This New Covenant is similar to the covenant God made with Abraham. God swore by Himself because there was no one greater than Him to be the witness (Hebrews 6:13-14). In Abrahamic's covenant, Abraham was NOT involved in cutting the covenant. God cut the covenant with Himself! (Genesis 15:12-18)

Similarly, in the New Covenant, we were NOT involved! **God cut the covenant with His Son Jesus.** Jesus was the perfect sacrifice. Because you and I are not involved in the covenant, there is nothing we can do to break that covenant. Now that you and I are IN Christ (Colossians 3:3; 1 Corinthians 1:30), we get the privilege to enjoy the covenant benefits.

Why is it important to know this? **There is NOTHING that can hinder us from receiving the benefits of the New Covenant, which includes healing**.

The redemptive works of Christ on the Cross have redeemed us to the position we had in the beginning. Now God looks at us justified (Romans 5:1; 1 Corinthians 6:11) – 'just as if we have never sinned before'. And if you have never sinned before, you can never suffer the effects of sin.

Disclaimer: I am not saying that you have never sinned before in reality. I am referring to your position in Christ. Because of Jesus' perfect sacrifice, your life is hidden in Him when you put your trust in Him (Colossians 3:3). God now sees you cleansed, sanctified, whole, AS IF you have never sinned before.

*And the Lord God formed man of the dust of the ground, and **breathed** into his nostrils the breath of life; and man became a living being.* - Genesis 2:7

At creation, God breathed life into the created Man. It was His Spirit imparted to Man. The word for 'breathed' in Hebrew is '*naphach*'.

After Jesus rose from the dead, He appeared to His disciples and breathed on them.

*And when He had said this, He **breathed** on them, and said to them, "Receive the **Holy Spirit**.* - John 20:22

The word 'breathed' used in John 20:22 is the Greek word '*emphusaó*'. This word is the first and only time it appears in the whole of the New Testament. If you look at the Septuagint (the Greek translation of the Hebrew Scriptures), 'emphusao' is the **<u>exact same word</u>** used for the word 'breathed' in Genesis 2:7.

καὶ ἔπλασεν ὁ Θεὸς τὸν ἄνθρωπον, χοῦν ἀπὸ τῆς γῆς, καὶ **ἐνεφύσησεν** εἰς τὸ πρόσωπον αὐτοῦ πνοὴν ζωῆς, καὶ ἐγένετο ὁ ἄνθρωπος εἰς ψυχὴν ζῶσαν. - Genesis 2:7 (The Septuagint)

καὶ τοῦτο εἰπὼν **ἐνεφύσησεν** καὶ λέγει αὐτοῖς· Λάβετε πνεῦμα ἅγιον· - John 20:22 (Greek Bible)

ἐνεφύσησεν = emphusao, which is translated as **'breathed'** in English!

At Redemption, Jesus breathed the Spirit of God (Holy Spirit) into fallen men, to redeem them back to the place BEFORE the Fall at Creation. What does that mean? We can now walk in the kind of health that Adam had! **Herein lies the secret to divine health ------- believing in the Redemptive works of Jesus Christ on the Cross**. It is perfectly perfect and completely complete! We have been redeemed from every sickness, disease, curse, virus, bacteria, and every form of death!

Healing Is In The Redemption

Unlike what some believe, healing is actually not in the Atonement. Healing is in the **Redemption!** In Atonement, sins were covered but not removed (Leviticus 16; Hebrews 10:1-4,11). In Redemption, sins were removed (Hebrews 10:12-18) so that we are redeemed!

The first compound name that God revealed to Israel after they came out of Egypt (bondage and sin) is Jehovah Rapha (Exodus 15:26) ------ which means 'I AM the Lord who heals you or makes you whole'.

*Now when they came to Marah, they could not drink the waters of Marah, for they were **bitter**. Therefore the name of it was called Marah. And the people complained against Moses, saying, "What shall* *we drink?" So he cried out to the Lord, and the **Lord showed him a tree**. When **he cast it into the waters, the waters were made sweet**.* - Exodus 15:23-25

The Old Covenant is New Covenant concealed, while the New Covenant is Old Covenant revealed. When the tree was cast into the bitter waters, they became sweet. The curse of bitterness was reversed! Right after that, God revealed Himself as Jehovah Rapha.

This points to the Redemption of Christ that is to come.

*Christ has **redeemed us from the curse of the law**, having become a curse for us (for it is written, "Cursed is everyone who hangs on a **tree")**. - Galatians 3:13*

Sickness is a curse (Deuteronomy 28:58-61). And we have been redeemed from that curse! Every healing, therefore, is a **confirmation** of Redemption!

Life In The Spirit

At Redemption, Jesus breathed the Spirit of God into men, and this is the same Spirit that raised Him from the dead.

*But if the Spirit of Him who raised Jesus from the dead dwells in you, He who raised Christ from the dead will also **give life to your mortal bodies through His Spirit who dwells in you**. - Romans 8:11*

Now that you and I have the Spirit of God who raised Jesus from the dead dwelling in us, the same life of God is within us. The life of God does not co-exist with sickness. The latter must die in the presence of divine life.

Some of you may wonder, "*Why am I not experiencing that? Why is sickness still in my body?*"

Do you believe in the Redemption of Christ?

According to your faith let it be to you. - Matthew 9:29

What you believe will ultimately be what you receive. If you believe in the Redemptive works of Christ, you will see your healing.

*For assuredly, I say to you, whoever says to this mountain, 'Be removed and be cast into the sea,' and **does not doubt in his heart, but** **believes** that those things he says will be done, **he will have whatever he says**. Therefore I say to you, whatever things you ask when you pray, **believe** **that you receive them, and you will have them**.* - Mark 11:23-24

People often say, "*I have prayed so many times, but I still don't see results/manifestations.*" Well, contrary to many teachings, prayer doesn't get you the result or manifestation. **Believing does**. You don't receive because you pray. You receive **because you believe**. There is a difference between praying because you are desperate, and praying because you believe. Most people do the former. But when you get into the Word and allow the Word to get into you, you will do the latter ------ **BELIEVE!**

Here is a testimony from **John G Lake**, the late American healing minister in the 19th-20th century. He was probably the most effective healing minister up to date. I'm sharing his testimony because it uses the same principle ---- the Spirit of Life in us!

"And because we were in contact with the Spirit of life, I and a little Dutch fellow with me went out and buried many of the people who had died from the bubonic plague. We went into the homes and carried them out, dug the graves and put them in. Sometimes we would put three or four in one grave. We never took the disease. Why? Because of the knowledge that the law of life in Christ Jesus protects us. That law was working. Because of the fact that a man by that action of his will, puts himself purposely in contact with God, faith takes possession of his heart, and the condition of his nature is changed. Instead of being fearful, he is full of faith. Instead of being absorbent and drawing everything to himself, his spirit repels sickness and disease. The Spirit of Christ Jesus flows through the whole being and emanates through the hands, the heart, and from every pore of the body.

During that great plague that I mentioned, they sent a government ship with supplies and corps of doctors. One of the doctors sent for me, and said, "What have you been using to protect yourself? Our corps has this preventative and that, which we use as protection, but we concluded that if a man could stay on the ground as you have and keep ministering to the sick and burying the dead, you must have a secret. What is it?"

I answered, "Brother that is the 'law of the Spirit of life in Christ Jesus.' I believe that just as long as I keep my soul in contact with the living God so that His Spirit is flowing into my soul and body, that no germ will ever attach itself to me, for the Spirit of God will kill it." He asked, "Don't you think that you had better use our preventatives?" I replied, "No, but doctor, I think that you would like to experiment with me. If you will go over to one of these dead people and take the foam that comes out of their lungs after death, then put it under the microscope you will see masses of living germs. You will find they are alive until a reasonable time after a man is dead. You can fill my hand with them and I will keep it under the microscope, and instead of these germs remaining alive, they will die instantly." They tried it and found it was true. They questioned, "What is that?" I replied, "That is 'the law of the Spirit of life in Christ Jesus.' When a man's spirit and a man's body are filled with the blessed presence of God, it oozes out of the pores of your flesh and kills the germs." - John G Lake, the bubonic plague in South Africa in the year 1908

Healing is in the Redemption of Christ. Because of Jesus' finished works, healing is freely given to you!

Believing Jesus As Your Personal Redeemer

Today, if you have not placed your trust in Jesus personally as your Redeemer, He can still heal you completely. But I would like to encourage you to take a step of faith and believe in Him ---- because He loves you and He is GOOD!

I deeply apologize, on behalf of the Christians, who have misrepresented who Jesus is. That includes me in the past. I am sorry that as Christians, we do not always live our lives in a way that represents Jesus fully. We preach a lot but we don't live what we preach. We have said and done things that hurt you. We have handled situations without integrity and basic morals. That is not who God has created us to be. And that is certainly not like Jesus. By His grace, we will live right, because He has put righteousness in us. Many of us simply do not understand and/or realize that He has already empowered us to walk in love, holiness, and high moral standards. As a result of the lack of understanding, we fail to live like Christians -------- the representation of Jesus Christ.

Having said that, believing in Jesus is a personal decision. Let not other Christians affect your decision. They don't necessarily represent Jesus. The clearest representation can be found in the Bible -------- The Gospel of Matthew, Mark, Luke and John. You can read them and discover who Jesus really is. You will realize Jesus is full of love and grace.

Christianity is not a religion. In religions, it's all about doing. If you do good, you get good. Otherwise, you get bad karma (retribution). In Christianity, it's all **DONE** -------- by Jesus Christ, God's beloved Son (John 3:16). In religions, men try to get to gods through good works and moral behaviors. In Christianity, God sought men. He came to us personally. Because there is no way in which we could get to Him by our own deeds and efforts. He created us, therefore, only He knows how to bring us back to Him.

When God created the world, He created men and women in His image (Genesis 1:26). We were His sons and daughters to begin with. Yet due to sin, we fell short of His standard (Romans 3:23), because we lost the nature within us to live right and do right (Romans 5:12). By the grace and the goodness of God, He came from heaven to earth and lived as a perfect Man without sin, in order to redeem imperfect men and women like you and me. Jesus, fully God, came from heaven to earth, to live as a Man so that He could reconcile you and me back into the relationship we were meant to have with God. We were lost. Now we can all be found by Him, **by returning to Him**.

Jesus didn't die just for our sin. **He died for our value.** The Cross is not just a revelation of our sin. More importantly, **the Cross is a revelation of our sonship**. Jesus died to restore our identity and our value as sons and daughters of the Most High God. He died for the lost. He came to seek and to save that which was lost. The Gospel is the redemption of the lost! To be lost means that we were in the right place to begin with ------- as sons and daughters of God. Jesus came to reconcile us back to that place. Only a broken relationship requires reconciliation. In other words, men and women were created originally to be in a relationship with God.

Jesus' life on earth was perfect. He healed the sick, cleansed the leper, raised the dead and cast out demons. He preached the Good News of who God is, desiring that people return to God. He went through severe persecution by those who rejected His message -------- He suffered betrayal, pain, rejection and abandonment from His loved ones; He took the whipping; He was nailed to the Cross.

On the Cross, Jesus was marred beyond human recognition. His bones were exposed (Psalm 22:17) because He was whipped so severely that His body was torn. The Roman whip comes with several strands, each about three feet long. Each strand is weighted with pieces of bones, metals and glasses. One single lash is likened to that of a shotgun's blast. It is so powerful that it rips open the flesh, severing layers of tissue and muscle. One lash would require 180 stitches to close up the wound. Jesus received more than 40 lashes, because He was whipped by the Romans, not the Jews. Some scholars believed that Jesus took more than 100 lashes such that He had no strength to carry His Cross on the road to Calvary.

If you think this is bad enough, it was not. They put a crown of thorns on Jesus' head, piercing through His flesh and causing even more blood to flow out. Not only that, they put a purple robe on Him. If you are already bleeding all over your body, with your flesh mostly gone and your bones fully exposed, the robe will stick to your body. In the later part, they removed the robe from Jesus' body. That resulted in extreme, intense and burning pain. But the Bible says that Jesus was thinking of us with love and joy. *"For the joy that was set before Him endured the Cross."* (Hebrews 12:2)

On the Cross, Jesus couldn't be recognized as a human. It was beyond human recognition (Isaiah 52:14). He went through this, so that you and I can have God's everlasting recognition. On the Cross, He lost His identity for a moment. He was forsaken as God's beloved and begotten Son (John 3:16), so that today, **you and I can never be forsaken**, and that **our identity can be restored as sons and daughters of God**. On the Cross, Jesus cried, *"My God, My God, why have You forsaken Me"*, so that today, you and I can say, *"**My Father, My Father, You never leave me nor forsake me.**"* You and I are God's beloved sons and daughters.

On the Cross, **God removed our sin and restored our value**. God forgave every single person through Jesus (2 Corinthians 5:19; Colossians 1:20). Jesus didn't go to the Cross just for Christians. He went to the Cross for the world! He wiped away our past and our mistakes, so that we can have a brand new start ------- **a brand new chance and a brand new life** to live differently. He wants to give you peace, joy, hope and abundance.

Will you return to Him who loves you unconditionally?

Will you say "Yes" to Him?

It is simple. You can simply say **"Yes"** to Him right now. Or you can say, "**I believe.**" He is God. He hears you wherever you are. You can also say, "*Thank You Jesus. I believe You died on the Cross for my sin and my value. You rose again and went back to heaven. Today, I return to You. I am coming back as your son (or daughter). Show me how to live in and through You.*"

If you have taken the step to believe in Jesus, I welcome you back to the family of God!

Do get connected with a community of believers (Christians) wherever you are, so that they can help you with this amazing journey!

Chapter 2:
The Great Hindrance

Many good and sincere believers think that if they don't receive healing, there must be some reasons or hindrances. As mentioned in Chapter 1, we must not interpret who God is based on our reasons and experiences. Don't even base it on what you hear from the pulpit. It must be based on who Jesus is and His finished works.

God's Will For Healing Was Established 2000 Years Ago

God is not changing His mind on healing. He never ever changes. If God only healed in the Gospel and not today, He has to change His name to "I WAS" instead of "I AM."

One of the clearest truths is established in Isaiah 53.

*Surely He has borne our **griefs** and carried our **sorrows**; yet we esteemed Him stricken, smitten by God, and afflicted. But He was wounded for our transgressions, He was bruised for our iniquities; the chastisement for our peace was upon Him, and **by His stripes we are healed**.* - Isaiah 53:4-5

The Hebrew word for 'griefs' is 'choli', which literally means '**sickness**.' The Hebrew word for 'sorrows' is 'makob', which literally means '**pain**.'

You can translate Isaiah 53:4 as '*Surely He has borne our **sickness** and carried our **pain**; yet we esteemed Him stricken, smitten by God, and afflicted.*'

In fact, we can let Scriptures interpret Scriptures to drive this truth deeper.

*When evening had come, they brought to Him many who were demon-possessed. And He cast out the spirits with a word, and **healed all who were sick, that it might be fulfilled which was spoken by***

Isaiah the prophet, saying: *"He Himself took our **infirmities** and bore our **sicknesses**."* - Matthew 8:16-17

Jesus healed ALL who were sick to confirm what Isaiah said in Isaiah 53:4. *'He Himself took our infirmities and bore our sicknesses.'* The Gospel interchanged the word 'griefs' and 'sorrows' in Isaiah 53:4 with 'infirmities' and 'sicknesses'. Nothing can be clearer than this!

*Surely He has borne our **sickness** and carried our **pain**...* - Isaiah 53:4

The reason why God inspired the author to write the word '**Surely**' is to assure us and give us the confidence that it is God's will to heal us! He knew that we would doubt in this area. What a loving Father we have!

*But He was wounded for **our transgressions**, He was bruised for **our iniquities**; the chastisement for our peace was upon Him, and **by His stripes we are healed**.* - Isaiah 53:5

When God talks about forgiveness of our sins, He also talks about healing (Psalm 103:1-3; Isaiah 53:4-12; Matthew 9:1-8). By the same token that He **bore our sins**, He also **bore our sicknesses and diseases**.

*Surely He has **borne** our griefs (sickness)...* - Isaiah 53:4 (emphasis added)

*And He **bore** the sin of many...* - Isaiah 53:12

In the same chapter of Isaiah, the word 'bore' was used twice. In Hebrew, it is the word '**nasa**' for both passages. 'Nasa' has the connotation of 'carrying'. It was used for both sickness and sin. When

Jesus bore our sin, He also bore our sicknesses and diseases. He didn't 'carry' one without the other. He carried **BOTH** in His body.

God has to put the word **'surely'** for Isaiah 53:4, because He probably knew that we would have difficulty believing that just as He has forgiven all our sins (salvation), He has healed us from all our sicknesses.

In fact, the word 'salvation' comes from the root word **'sozo'**, which means 'saved, healed, delivered, protected, preserved, made whole, kept safe and sound'. Salvation does not only refer to the saving of one's spirit, it includes physical and emotional healing, deliverance and much more! God didn't mean for us to compartmentalize what salvation is. **Salvation means complete wholeness** (sozo)! Read also in Mark 5:34; Luke 17:19; Mark 10:52.

Therefore He is also able to **save to the uttermost** *those who come to God through Him...* - Hebrews 7:25

The word 'save' here is the same Greek word **'sozo'**, which means wholeness! So if God can save to the uttermost, it also means that **God is able to heal to the uttermost** ------ no matter what kind of sickness you are going through!

What kind of sickness are you going through? Know that God loves you so much that He has given His Son, so that you can be healed!

In Isaiah 53:5, it says 'by His stripes we **are** healed.' That was Isaiah prophesying 800 years before Christ was born. When Christ took the stripes (John 19:1), the prophecy was fulfilled.

Who Himself bore our sins in His own body on the tree, that we, having died to sins, might live for righteousness - by whose stripes you **were healed**. - 1 Peter 2:24

Did you notice that the healing has been changed to past tense ('were') in 1 Peter 2:24, instead of the present tense ('are') in Isaiah 53:5?

This indicates that healing was established when Jesus received the stripes. He took every sickness and bore every pain in His body 2000 years ago. In God's perspective, healing is a done deal. **God's will and His timing to heal you have long been established 2000 years ago when Jesus died!**

If the event (Jesus' stripes) happened 2000 years ago, it also means that there is no appointed timing for you to be healed, just as there is no appointed timing for you to be forgiven.

Today, you no longer need to pray, "*God, is it not yet Your timing to heal me? I will wait.*" God's timing was established 2000 years ago. This is why 1 Peter 2:24 says that 'by His stripes you **WERE** healed.'

Today, you no longer need to pray, "*God, if it is Your will, heal me. Yet not my will, but Yours be done.*" This kind of prayer completely ignores Jesus' sacrifice and treats it as though Jesus died in vain!

Today, you can be fully certain and confident that it is **God's will** and **His timing** for you **to be healed EVERY SINGLE TIME!** You don't need His permission. You don't need to ask Him. Healing has been released for you. The gift has been given 2000 years ago. Now it is on your end to simply **BELIEVE** and **RECEIVE**.

There Is No Hindrance To Your Healing

The only hindrance to healing is to believe that there is a possible hindrance to your healing.

I'm going to share a list of religious traditions that have been taught widely when someone doesn't get healed. These are sacred cows that should be destroyed. By removing these wrong beliefs in your heart, you are ready to receive healing.

*Beware lest anyone cheat you through philosophy and empty deceit, **according to the tradition of men**, according to the basic principles of the world, and **not according to Christ**. - Colossians 2:8*

*...making the word of God of no effect **through your tradition** which you have handed down. - Mark 7:13*

If we believe in traditions and not what Christ has said and done, we are believing in a lie. Believing in a lie prevents us from experiencing the breakthrough God has already given to us. For example, if you believe that you need anointing oil in order to receive healing, you won't be healed when there is no anointing oil. Why? Because you believe in a lie. It's done according to your belief (Matthew 9:29).

IMPORTANT: The only hindrance to healing is when you believe there can be hindrances to healing.

If salvation is by grace through faith in Christ alone, then healing is the same ------- healing is by grace through faith in Christ alone. **Don't put any qualification on healing that Jesus didn't!** If God did not spare His beloved, treasured and begotten Son, but gave Him up for us all (Romans 8:32), how would He not also with Him, **freely and graciously give us ALL THINGS, which include healing?!**

The saving of our spirit requires the death of God's Son, Jesus. The healing of our body requires the stripes of Jesus. From this comparison, it seems to require a 'greater' effort to save our spirit. And if God has freely given us the 'greater', He will surely give us the 'lesser'.

If we can trust Him for what is 'greater' (like salvation) ------ bringing us to heaven, why can't we trust Him for what is 'lesser' ------- healing of our body on earth? It has to do with our perception.

Destroying Sacred Cows

1) I'm not healed because God is still teaching me through this sickness

If you were a parent, would you use sickness to teach your children? *"Hey son, are you having a fever? That's good for you. Don't go to the doctor. I want you to first learn about patience and humility."* That's ridiculous!

We may laugh it off. But if we, as imperfect parents won't do that, how could we think of God, the Perfect Father doing that to us?

God doesn't teach us by using sickness. He teaches us primarily **by His Word**.

*I am the true vine, and My Father is the vinedresser. Every branch in Me that does not bear fruit He takes away; and every branch that bears fruit He **prunes**, that it may bear more fruit. You are already **clean** because of the word which I have spoken to you. - John 15:1-3*

Some think that when God prunes you to grow in character, He will give you sickness or pain. Nothing is further from the truth. The word

28

'prune' and the word 'clean' actually come from the same root word 'katharus', which means 'to cleanse'. In other words, you can read the above passage like this --- '*Every branch in Me that bears fruit He prunes, that it may bear more fruit. You are already pruned **because of the word** which I have spoken to you.*'

God primarily teaches by His Word!

*All Scripture is God-breathed and is useful for **teaching**, rebuking, correcting and training in righteousness...* - 2 Tim 3:16

2) What about Job? He suffered from sickness.

Firstly, sickness is NOT part of suffering (James 5:13-14). I will share more on this in sacred cow number 7.

Secondly, Job did not have a clear revelation of who God is (Job 42:5) in those days. He didn't even have a proper understanding of who satan is (John 8:44; 10:10). Only Jesus came to reveal the exact revelation of who God is (John 1:18; 14:9; Hebrews 1:3).

Thirdly, not everything written about God is true in the book of Job (Job 1:21; 13:15; 19:6; 19:21; 33:8-10).

*"Naked I came from my mother's womb, and naked shall I return there. The Lord gave, and the **Lord has taken away**; blessed be the name of the Lord."* - Job 1:21

This is a popular verse that Christians like to quote, and even sing in worship songs. They think it's a holy passage to meditate and talk about. This sacred cow has to be killed.

What Job said about God is wrong. It is not who God is. The Lord indeed gives, but He does **NOT** take away. The one who takes away, the one who steals, kills and destroys is the enemy (John 10:10). God is the Giver of Life (Psalm 36:8-9). Jesus came to give life, and life more abundantly. Never once did you see Jesus taking away life and/or blessings throughout the books of the Gospel. He is the Resurrection and the Life (John 11:25). He is the Way, the Truth and the Life (John 14:6).

Not every worship song we sing is biblical. Some have to be removed from our worship song list.

It is clear that satan was the one who afflicted Job (Job 1:12). However, we must understand the Hebrew mindset. In those days, the Hebrew writers did not have a clear revelation of God and satan. In fact, the Hebrew Bible did not record the proper name of 'Satan' (with a capital S). They thought that there was no devil and demons. Evil and suffering in their worldview had one original source: God Himself. They believed that God alone controlled all events (including satan) and was responsible for all conditions within creation, whether good or evil. If you read the Old Testament, you will read stuff like 'an evil spirit from the Lord', 'I form the light and create darkness, I make peace and create calamity', etc. It is, therefore, important, to understand the context of those writings and rightly divide the Word in the light of Christ and His finished works ---------- that is the foundation of who God truly is. There is a lot to cover on bible interpretations, understanding the various covenants in the Bible, approaches in reading the Old Testament, etc. But that's not the purpose of this manual. We have to focus on healing.

Job, in like manner, thought that it was God who took away his family, possessions and health, when the reality is that satan was the one who stole, killed and destroyed.

We must understand that when Man fell and gave the authority of dominion on earth to satan (Luke 4:6), the latter could have access to God anytime (Job 1:6-7). The world lies in his power (1 John 5:19) because they don't know that Jesus has taken back the authority (Matthew 28:18). As believers, we do know, and therefore, Job is not our example. Jesus is.

Job was living in a time when Jesus had not yet come. The authority of dominion on earth was with satan. When God said in Job 1:12, '*Behold, all that he has is in your power; only do not lay a hand on his person*', God was simply stating the fact that satan had all the power to destroy Job (1 John 5:19; John 10:10). But God did not allow satan to touch Job's life. '*Do not lay a hand on his person*' is simply God's divine protection over Job's life.

Note: I like to spell satan in small letters, because I think he is very small as compared to God.

Didn't God give satan permission to harm Job?

*Then the Lord said to Satan, "**Have you considered** My servant Job, that there is none like him on the earth, a blameless and upright man, one who fears God and shuns evil?" - Job 1:8*

*Then the Lord said to Satan, "**Have you considered** My servant Job, that there is none like him on the earth, a blameless and upright man, one who fears God and shuns evil? And still he holds fast to his* *integrity, although you incited Me against him, to destroy him without cause."* - Job 2:3

The English translation is not always the best translation. In Hebrew, the phrase 'have you considered' is actually **'set your mind or heart towards'**. The Young's Literal Translation actually translated the verse better.

*And Jehovah saith unto the Adversary, '**Hast thou set thy heart against** My servant Job because there is none like him in the land, a man perfect and upright, fearing God, and turning aside from evil?' -* Job 1:8 (YLT)

*And Jehovah saith unto the Adversary, '**Hast thou set thy heart** unto My servant Job because there is none like him in the land, a man perfect and upright, fearing God and turning aside from evil? and still he is keeping hold on his integrity, and thou dost move Me against him to swallow him up for nought!' -* Job 2:3 (YLT)

This has a totally different meaning from the normal English translations. God wasn't giving satan permission to harm Job. God was simply stating the fact because He is all-knowing --------- satan already set his heart against Job. He had planned in his mind to attack Job and destroy his family, possessions and health.

God correctly said to satan, *"you incited Me against him..."* Because the devil is the accuser of the brethren (Zechariah 3:1-2; Revelation 12:10). He didn't approach God to get permission. He didn't need any permission because he already held the authority (1 John 5:19). He approached God simply to accuse Job (Job 1:9-11; 2:4-5) and went ahead to destroy him.

In a nutshell, **satan was the one who afflicted Job, and God was the One who protected his life** (Job 1:12; 2:6), restored and blessed him (Job 42:10-12).

The book of Job is not meant to teach the theology of suffering. It is meant to teach on perseverance during trials, while believing God for His faithful deliverance.

*You have heard of the **perseverance** of Job and seen **the end intended by the Lord**—that the **Lord is very compassionate and merciful**.* - James 5:11

3) It is not God's timing for me to be healed yet

We have established this earlier in Chapter 2. God's will and His timing for you to be healed were long established 2000 years ago when Jesus died (Isaiah 53:4-5; 1 Peter 2:24). From that time onward, it is always God's timing for you to be healed and made whole **NOW**!

4) I am not healed because of generational curses and/or sins

People who teach about generational curses or sins usually quote the verses from the Old Testament such as Exodus 34:6-7; Numbers 14:18; Deuteronomy 5:9; etc. You cannot find them in the New Testament.

Again, as mentioned before, if you believe that, it shall be done according to your belief.

The truth is that we are in Christ ------ the New Covenant (Jeremiah 31:29-31; Hebrews 8:12-13). Therefore, there is no generational curse or sin when you are IN Christ. Your past generation is Christ and Christ alone!

If anyone wants to repent for the sins of their past generations, they should do so all the way back to Adam!

*For I will be merciful to their unrighteousness, and their sins and their lawless deeds **I will remember no more**. In that He says, "**A new covenant**," He has made the first obsolete.* - Hebrews 8:12-13

*Christ has **redeemed** us from the curse of the law...* - Galatians 3:13

The word 'redeemed' comes from the root word 'completely out from'. We are **completely out from** generational sins and curses the moment we put our trust in Jesus!

What about John 9?

*And His disciples asked Him, saying, "Rabbi, who sinned, this man **or his parents**, that he was born blind?" Jesus answered, "Neither this man nor his parents sinned, **but that the works of God should be revealed in him**.* - John 9:2-3

In the Jewish culture, they believed that a person's sickness is a result of divine-mandated punishment, either due to his own sin, or the sin of his family. This was why the disciples asked the question. Jesus answered, "**Neither**... *but that the works of God should be revealed in him.*"

Sickness is not necessarily caused by sin. It could be an attack of the enemy; it could be other people's bad choices affecting you.

Whatever the cause might be, Jesus wasn't concerned with the root issue at all! He didn't need to dig out the past or so-called root causes. He was there to **BE THE ANSWER**! He was there to be the solution.

He presented the answer ----- healing (John 9:7) and the man was completely healed!

Throughout the Gospel books, Jesus never asked anyone to repent of his parents' sins or his own sins, in order to be healed. The church today has gotten it backward. Jesus never placed a qualification for someone to be healed. To think that you are qualified to be healed already disqualifies you from the grace of God.

If we can say a general "*Be healed"* in a healing meeting with masses and see people healed, why do we need to go into the specifics and root causes when we minister to an individual? If we need to dig out the past or root causes from someone who is sick in order to minister healing, we obviously do not carry the Answer Jesus has!

Jesus is the same yesterday, today and forever. He doesn't need to know what your past generations did, before He can heal you. **He is here to be your solution. He is the Healer!**

Note: The whole of the New Testament epistles does not record any single thing about generational curses or sins. On the contrary, it imparts the truth of who you are (2 Corinthians 5:17; Colossians 3:3; Galatians 2:20; Romans 6:3-4). You are a new creation! Stop looking to the past. Start looking to Jesus, the Author and the Finisher of your faith! (Hebrews 12:2).

5) I need an atmosphere of healing to be healed

In the Old Covenant, the presence of God was outside of the people (Exodus 13:21; 33:14).

In the New Covenant, the presence of God is **IN** us (John 14:16-18; Colossians 1:27; Acts 2:1-4).

We are not looking outward for healing. We are looking within for health (Romans 8:11). The kingdom of God is where God reigns and where He reigns, there is no sickness (Matthew 12:28). Guess where this kingdom of God is? It's right **WITHIN** you (Luke 12:32; 17:21).

*Now Peter and John went up together to the temple at the **hour of prayer**, the ninth hour.* - Acts 3:1

Peter and John were going to the temple to pray. They were not 'prayed up' yet. They hadn't gone into an atmosphere (or some say 'corporate anointing') of healing. They were not fasting. They were not doing anything. But the Scriptures tell us that they healed the lame man (Acts 3:1-8) while they were going to the temple to pray.

Peter gave the answer when the crowd thought that he had some special powers to heal the lame man. He said in Acts 3:16 - *"And His name, through **faith in His name**, has made this man strong."*

Healing is solely by grace through faith in Jesus alone!

6) If I believe in healing, I must not go to the doctor or take any medication

The Gospel didn't record any instance on the use of medication. However, in the epistles, we see that Paul told Timothy to use some wine for his stomach problem.

No longer drink only water, but use a little wine for your stomach's sake and your frequent infirmities. - 1 Timothy 5:23

In those days, it was common for the Romans to mix wine in water before they drank, because of the contamination of water, which caused stomach issues. This passage has been used by skeptics to say that healing didn't take place for Timothy when Paul, his spiritual father, ministered to him. Nothing is further from the truth. We cannot interpret the Word by omission. We cannot conclude what is not written in the Scriptures. We must interpret the Word based on Jesus, who is the Word made flesh (John 1:14). The fundamental way for interpretation is to focus on the explicit, instead of the implicit. We need to let what is clear interpret what is unclear.

Jesus healed ALL who came to Him. **Even the disciples healed ALL who came to them** (Acts 5:16; 28:9). Healing is unquestionably the will and desire of God!

It is more likely that Timothy was living in a condition where water contamination was prevalent. That resulted in his frequent stomach issues. Paul advised him to mix the water with wine, which served to purify stagnant water sources and make them drinkable.

In today's context, I believe that we shouldn't go to the extreme and stop anyone from the use of medication. We should lift up and encourage one another, instead of saying things that put them under condemnation. Not everyone is walking at the same level of conviction concerning healing and health.

But even as we are using medication, our focus should always be on Jesus. Our trust is upon Him who heals, instead of the doctor or the medication. God can and will still heal us while we are taking the medication. When you are made whole, your body will tell you when to stop the medication.

Unless your conviction tells you otherwise, you can continue the medication and at the same time, receive healing from Jesus.

7) I still have sin in my life. Therefore, I cannot be healed

You cannot find any Scripture in the New Testament on this sacred cow.

In fact, everyone whom Jesus healed in the four books of the Gospel was sinners. They were living in sin, and they knew nothing about holy living. They were not born again!

Jesus healed a lame man who was living in sin (John 5:1-14), **BEFORE** telling him not to sin again.

*The **goodness** of God leads you to repentance.* - Romans 2:4

It is the goodness (which includes healing) of God that leads us to repentance. Don't get it the other way round. If God sent His Son to die for your sins when you were still a sinner (Romans 5:6) and an enemy of God (Romans 5:8), why would He withhold the 'lesser' (healing) from you (Romans 8:32)?

IMPORTANT: While sin may cause you to be sick, sin does **NOT** hinder nor stop God from healing you!

What about James 5:16? It says, *"Confess your trespasses to one another, and pray for one another, that you may be healed."*

Remember, a text without the context will always be a pretext for a prooftext. This has nothing to do with physical healing. Let's read the earlier verses.

*Is anyone among you **suffering**? Let him pray. Is anyone cheerful? Let him sing psalms. Is anyone among you **sick**? Let him call for the elders of the church, and let them pray over him, anointing* *him with oil in the name of the Lord. And the prayer of **faith** will save the sick, and the Lord will raise him up. **And if he has committed sins**, he will be forgiven.* - James 5:13-15

I highlighted the words intentionally to show you how we can easily interpret the passage. Notice, suffering and sickness are two separate issues! In fact, sickness is not part of a Christian's suffering. **Don't suffer for what Jesus already paid to give us on the Cross.** His body was broken so that our bodies can be made whole.

The only Christian suffering that is biblical and promised is persecution (2 Timothy 3:12; 2 Corinthians 12:10; Romans 5:1-5).

James was clear in his writing that suffering and sickness are separate issues altogether. For sickness, he taught the church to get the elders to minister healing! It is the responsibility of elders. Elders are supposed to have faith (though it is not always the case in today's churches) for the sick to be healed.

The word 'prayer' used in this verse is different from the usual word used in many parts of the Bible. In fact, it is only used in this context once in this passage throughout the whole of the New Testament. It speaks of a promise; a vow. As believers, we don't pray from earth to heaven as if we need to beg God for healing. We pray from heaven to heaven (Ephesians 2:6). We can declare that healing is done. That's the prayer of faith!

It is faith in Christ that heals the sick (Mark 11:22-24; Acts 3:16; see Page 18-19 again).

Look at James 5:13-15 again. James wrote, '**And if he has committed sins**, *he will be forgiven.*' Does this verse come before the sick is healed, or after the sick is healed? **AFTER!**

The sick is healed **whether** he has committed sins or not. Healing is always released before we talk about repentance. It is the goodness of God that leads one to repentance! (Romans 2:4)

Now you can look at James 5:16 in context, *"Confess your **trespasses** to one another, and pray for one another, that you may be healed."*

Since James had already given instructions to handle suffering and sickness (James 5:13-15), verse 16 cannot be talking about sickness again!

The word 'trespasses' in Greek is the word 'paraptoma', which can be translated as 'fault' or 'offense'. You can read it like this, *"Confess your faults/offenses to one another, and pray for one another, that you may be healed."*

This is similar to the words of Jesus in the Gospel book.

*Moreover if your brother sins against you, go and tell him **his fault between you and him alone**. If he hears you, you have gained your brother.* - Matthew 18:15

The only reason why you need to confess your faults and offenses to one another is that you want the relationship to be healed and reconciled! When you confess your offenses against each other WITH each other, and when you pray for each other, you will be healed relationally. You gain a brother/sister. You gain a restored relationship.

*Then He began to rebuke the cities in which most of His mighty works had been done, **because they did not repent**.* - Matthew 11:20

Jesus did most of His miracles and healings in cities where the people did not repent. They were still in sin!

Sin doesn't stop God from healing you. It, however, may stop you from receiving from Him if you do not understand His goodness and mercy. In part 3 of this manual, **The Great Secret**, we will look into this deeper and establish the truth once and for all.

8) I need more healing anointing to be healed

Again, you can't find any Scriptures in the Bible that talk about this. This is often taught in the charismatic circles that are not grounded in the Word.

In the Old Covenant, the anointing of God did not abide in a person. It could come and go, and was often given based on the assignments in their lives ---- usually kings and prophets (1 Samuel 16:13-14; Leviticus 8:12).

Elisha asked for a double portion of Elijah's spirit (2 Kings 2:9). This has resulted in many preachers teaching that there is a double portion of anointing that you can ask God for. Some even teach that you can ask an anointed man to lay hand on you and impart a double portion of anointing.

First of all, we have to understand the context of the passage. The Hebrews understood the concept of succession. Under that culture, if you have two sons, the elder son gets a double portion of the inheritance that the father left behind. In other words, the elder son gets 2/3 while the younger son gets 1/3. If there are three sons, the eldest son gets 2/4, while the rest of the sons get 1/4 each. The eldest son will always receive a double portion of the father's inheritance, as compared to other sons in the family.

When Elisha asked for a double portion of Elijah's spirit, it was about desiring the right of the firstborn. The 'double portion' refers to Elijah's recognition of Elisha as his immediate successor and to treat him like a firstborn son.

Look at what Elisha cried out when Elijah was taken up.

*Then it happened, as they continued on and talked, that suddenly a chariot of fire appeared with horses of fire, and separated the two of them; and Elijah went up by a whirlwind into heaven. And Elisha saw it, and he cried out, "**My father, my father**, the chariot of Israel and its horsemen!" So he saw him no more. -* 2 Kings 2:12

Elisha simply requested to be Elijah's successor by asking for a double portion of his spirit. As his successor, Elisha would naturally have a 'greater' portion of inheritance than other prophets in his days. It certainly did not mean that Elisha had a double portion of anointing as compared to Elijah.

Some argued that Elisha indeed did more miracles than Elijah. Others reasoned that Elisha did twice as much.

Even if it was so, it merely confirmed what would happen in and through Christ. Remember, the Old Covenant contains types that simply foreshadow the New.

*Most assuredly, I say to you, he who believes in Me, the works that I do he will do also; and **greater works than these** he will do, because I go to My Father. -* John 14:12

Elijah was a type of Christ. Just as Christ went to the Father in heaven, Elijah was taken up to heaven. Just as Elisha did more miracles than Elijah, Jesus said that we would do **greater works** than what He did!

Does that mean that we have a double portion of Christ's anointing? Nothing is further from the truth.

In fact, **as believers of the New Covenant, we now have the fullness of God dwelling within us** (John 3:34; Colossians 2:9-10; 1 Corinthians 1:30). We have an anointing that abides and never leaves, and that anointing is the Holy Spirit!

*But **the anointing** which you have received from Him **abides in you**, and you do not need that anyone teach you; but as the **same anointing teaches you concerning all things**, and is true, and is not a lie, and just as it has taught you, you will abide in Him.* - 1 John 2:27

*But the Helper, the **Holy Spirit**, whom the Father will send in My name, He will **teach you all things**, and bring to your remembrance all things that I said to you.* - John 14:26

If the anointing points to the Holy Spirit, every single believer, including you and I, are equally anointed! However, if you believe in a lie ------ that other men and women of God are more anointed than you, then it shall be done according to your belief (Mathew 9:29).

The Holy Spirit is upon you BECAUSE you already are anointed as His sons and daughters (Luke 4:18). You are not anointed because the Holy Spirit comes upon you. On the contrary, the Holy Spirit is upon you because you are anointed!

Stop looking to the men of God at the pulpit. **Start looking to the God of Man who lives in you and died for you** ------ Jesus Christ ------- the Anointed One is **IN** you!

You don't need more healing anointing. You already have the fullness. You just need to believe more, that the anointing to heal is within you. As you destroy these religious traditions by believing in the truths that I show you, the anointing will become more and more evident in your life!

9) I cannot be healed because of an atmosphere of unbelief

I have heard of some healing ministers using the following passage to teach about the need to have an atmosphere of belief.

Now He could do no mighty work there, except that He laid His hands on a few sick people and healed them. And He marveled because of their unbelief. - Mark 6:5-6

Some teach that Jesus could not do any miracle because of the atmosphere of unbelief. Apparently, they believe that unbelief in the atmosphere can shut down Jesus' anointing and power to heal. They even conclude this with the passage where Jesus put everyone out of Jairus' house (Mark 5:40), for unbelief can prevent Jesus from raising the 12-year old girl from the dead.

Like I said before, **without context**, everything can be misinterpreted.

All things are **POSSIBLE** to Him who believes (Mark 9:23). If Jesus believes, how can anything stop healing from flowing? **Nothing is impossible for Jesus who believes!**

In Mark 6:5-6, Jesus laid His hands on a few sick people and healed them. It was either they managed to reach Jesus for healing or they simply couldn't really move away from Him in the synagogue. Because whomever He touched would surely be healed and made whole.

The whole context for the story in Mark 6:5-6 can be found in **Luke 4:16-30**. Compare it with Mark 6:1-6. It revealed the real reason why Jesus couldn't do mighty works there.

*So all those in the synagogue, when they heard these things, were filled with wrath, and rose up and **thrust Him out of the city**; and they led Him to the brow of the hill on which their city was built, that they might throw Him down over the cliff. Then passing through the midst of them, He went His way.* - Luke 4:28-30

Remember: We should always let Scripture interprets Scripture whenever it is possible. The Jews thrust Jesus out of the synagogue. They rejected Him. If you plan to heal the sick in a room, but you were rejected and thrust out of the room, it is obvious why you couldn't do miracles. Because nobody could come to you for healing!

It was not that Jesus couldn't heal the sick because of the presence of unbelief in the atmosphere (or in the hearts of people). It was because **He was literally chased out of the place**.

What about Jesus putting everyone out of the room before He raised Jairus' daughter from the dead? In fact, Peter did the same thing in Acts 9:40.

As I mentioned before, we cannot interpret the Scriptures based on omission ---- we cannot conclude what is not written in the Word. It must be inductive, instead of deductive. We can only conclude based on what is explicit.

Firstly, if you read the whole book of Acts, you will realize that it is a historical book and in it, contains progressive revelations of the New Covenant. Peter himself was progressively learning and growing (Acts 10:9-29). He could have simply followed Jesus because that was the only model he saw on raising a dead young girl.

*Then He came to the house of the ruler of the synagogue, and **saw a tumult and those who wept and wailed loudly**. When He came in, He said to them, "Why make this commotion and weep? The child is not dead, but sleeping."* - Mark 5:38-39

In the Jewish culture of those days, it was common to hire professional mourners at funerals. They would weep and wail loudly to remind everyone about the sadness and pain that is associated when someone passes on. It was very probable that Jesus simply wanted them to stop making the commotion in the room. And so, He put them all out of the room.

*Then He began to rebuke the cities in which **most of His mighty works** had been done, because they did not repent.* - Matthew 11:20

Contrary to popular religious beliefs, unbelief cannot stop Jesus from healing and doing miracles. He did most of His miracles in cities full of unbelief.

What you believe can crush every ounce of unbelief in the room.

10) Fasting gets me healed

This is one of the most religious sacred cows that should be killed! Nowhere in the New Covenant teaches you that fasting gets you ANYTHING.

Some will quote *"However, this kind does not go out except by prayer and fasting"* (Read Matthew 17:19-21) to teach that certain healing or deliverance requires fasting.

This verse, however, was NOT recorded in most of the early Greek manuscripts of the New Testament. Many scholars believe that it was added later by the scribes, after comparing with the other Gospel books. It is often concluded that the original Matthew writing did NOT have verse 21. Looking at Mark 9 will give us a clearer perspective. The Gospel of Mark was recorded much earlier than the Gospel of Matthew.

And He said to them, "This kind cannot come out by anything but prayer." - Mark 9:29

Apparently, fasting is NOT recorded in the verse. It is not in the Greek translation too.

So why was fasting added into Matthew 17:21? The Gospel of Matthew was written to the Jews. The Gospel of Mark was written to the Gentiles.

In those days, the Jewish culture understood fasting. It's part of their yearly practice under the Law (Leviticus 23:26-32). However, they did it without the understanding of what true fast really meant (Isaiah 58). It was probable that verse 21 was added later into the manuscripts to include fasting for the Jewish readers.

The Gentile readers (Roman Christians), whom the Gospel of Mark was mainly written to, had no practice on fasting. Mark must have recorded what Jesus said, *"This kind cannot come out by anything except prayer."*

Prayer simply refers to communion and intimacy. Does this mean that certain healing/deliverance requires intimate communion with God? We will talk more about this in Chapter 6.

What we need to establish here is that fasting is not the key to your healing. Fasting is not bending God's will to do ours. It doesn't bend His hands to do something. Fasting doesn't bring any increase in power, breakthrough or answered prayers. It doesn't even move God. Let me repeat. Fasting does not move God. Believing does (Matthew 21:22; Mark 11:23-24).

Fasting is simply a tool to move us (our fleshly desires) out of the way so that He can have His way. Fasting is one of the ways to bring us to a place of focus (1 Corinthians 7:5) so that we become conscious of His presence and power which **we ALREADY have in Christ** that we can walk in.

Do you have to fast? **The answer is no**. Mark 2:18-20 is clear. *"As long as they have the bridegroom with them, they cannot fast."*

Jesus was with the disciples, thus they didn't need to fast. But Jesus would go to the Cross, and the disciples would fast (an act of mourning). In fact, Jesus interchanged the word 'fast' with 'mourn' (Matthew 9:15). After Jesus resurrected, He gave His disciples the Holy Spirit, who *"will never leave you nor forsake you."* Where is the Bridegroom now? By the Spirit of Christ, He lives IN us and WITH us.

This destroys the religious sacred cow of the obligation to fast in the New Covenant. Jesus fasted in the old nature, so that you and I can feast in the new nature. We feast on His body and blood through communion (John 6:54-56).

Whether you fast or not, it is the fruit that counts. It is all about life transformation. It is about becoming Him who is love. I have been living a lifestyle of fasting until I learnt what it means to **live a fasted life**. A fasted life can be summarized in Galatians 2:20.

*I have been crucified with Christ. It is no longer I who live, **but Christ lives in me**. And the life which I now live in the flesh, **I live by faith in the Son of God**, who loved me and gave Himself for me.* - Galatians 2:20

Most of the reasons for fasting in our present day context are out of wrong motives and/or wrong understanding. To God, it's a zero even if you fast for 40 days. Fasting is one of the available tools that God has graciously given to us for the purpose of focus. Apart from fasting, there are other tools which you can use, such as worship music, tongues, soaking prayer, etc. Use whatever tool that helps you to grow in intimacy with Him.

There is no obligation to fast in the New Covenant. Besides, if you think that fasting can get you something that the Cross can't, then Jesus died in vain and you are still worshiping religion.

11) Someone ministered healing to me, but I don't have enough faith to be healed.

If anyone ministers healing to you and says this, "*You don't have enough faith. That's why you are not healed*", run far away from him or her. That is a lie from the pit of hell. This is a guilt trip that is not biblical.

Nothing is further from the truth. Jesus NEVER once said that to the sick. When He raised the dead (Mark 5:35-43; Luke 7:11-17; John 11:33-44), did the dead or their family have faith? No!

When Jesus healed Peter's mother-in-law who had a fever and was lying on the bed (Matthew 8:14-15), did she have faith? When Jesus healed the demon-possessed boy (Mark 9:24), did he and his father have faith? When Jesus healed the man with an infirmity of 38 years (John 5:7-8), did he have faith? By no means!

There are so many passages in the Bible to prove that Jesus didn't need the sick to have faith when He ministered healing to them. Jesus healed them not because of their faith, but because of who He is. He is Jehovah Rapha, the Healer!

When Peter and John walked to the Temple in Acts 3, they saw a lame man. The latter asked them for money. Peter said, *"Silver and gold I do not have, but what I do have I give to you. In the name of Jesus Christ of Nazareth, rise up and walk!"* The man was totally healed!

The lame man did not even ask for healing, but he still received healing. Here lies an important truth --------- you don't even need the sick's permission to minister healing to him and see him healed.

As you get ministered by others for healing, it has nothing to do with your faith. **Rest and receive in Jesus' name.**

12) I need a Rhema Word, not Logos to be healed.

There are some in the charismatic circles who believe that you need a rhema word to be healed. They often quote Romans 10:17.

*So then faith comes by hearing, and hearing by the **word** of God. -* Romans 10:17

'Rhema' is used for 'word' in Romans 10:17.

'Rhema' is often believed to be the spoken word of God, while 'Logos' is the written word of God or Jesus Himself.

I did a study on the words and found out that both words are interchangeable!

*And the Lord turned and looked at Peter. Then Peter remembered the **word** of the Lord, how He had said to him, "Before the rooster crows, you will deny Me three times." -* Luke 22:61

*And Peter remembered the **word** of Jesus who had said to him, "Before the rooster crows, you will deny Me three times." So he went out and wept bitterly. -* Matthew 26:75

'Rhema' was used for 'word' in Matthew, while 'Logos' was used for 'word' in Luke. They are interchangeable!

You can also compare Hebrews 4:12 (Logos) and Ephesians 6:17 (Rhema), where both passages describe the Word of God as a sword. Read also Hebrews 11:3 (Rhema) and 2 Peter 3:5 (Logos), where both passages talk about heavens and earth that were created by the word of God.

Not convinced? Read the following.

Having been born again, not of corruptible seed but incorruptible, through the **word** *(Logos)* **of God which lives and abides forever,** *because "All flesh is as grass, and all the glory of man as the flower of the grass. The grass withers, and its flower falls away, but the* **word** *(Rhema)* **of the Lord endures forever.**" - 1 Peter 2:23-25 (emphasis added)

Nowhere in the Bible tells you that 'Rhema' and 'Logo' are different. It is simply a religious mindset, a sacred cow that has to be destroyed!

"If you want to know God's will, read the Word. If you want to be led by the Spirit, do the Word." - Lester Sumrall, the late American evangelist (1913-1996)

You don't need a so-called 'Rhema' word to be healed. You don't need a 'now' word from God. Healing was already paid for 2000 years ago! You just need to believe in the perfect and complete work of Jesus. **By His stripes, you were and are healed!**

Chapter 3:

The Great Secret

The Gospel of Jesus Christ is simple. Healing is simple. So let's not make it complicated.

The Secret to Divine Healing

Jesus didn't pay for your healing on the Cross. He didn't do that on the Cross.

Understanding this is vital in unlocking the secret to your healing.

*But He was wounded for our transgressions, He was bruised for our iniquities; the chastisement for our peace was upon Him, and **by His stripes** we are healed. - Isaiah 53:5*

*Who Himself bore our sins in His own body on the tree, that we, having died to sins, might live for righteousness — **by whose stripes** you were healed. - 1 Peter 2:24*

Scriptures only point us to His stripes when it comes to healing.

The secret to divine healing, therefore, rests in the truth that **Jesus took the stripes** for you and me.

As such, we must understand what He took for us. In fact, the word 'stripes' in both Hebrew and Greek is translated as **a singular 'stripe'**. In those days, if the Roman whip causes many stripes on your body, it will be written as 'stripes.' However, if there is not a single inch of flesh left in your body that is not whipped, it will be written as a singular 'stripe'. Jesus was whipped by the Roman soldiers, who did not have to follow the Jewish law (39 stripes). He could have been whipped way MORE than 39 stripes (I can imagine 100 or more!), such that there was not even an inch of flesh left in His body!

This is why the Psalmist wrote, "*I can count all My bones.*" (Psalm 22:17)

Mel Gibson's movie 'The Passion of the Christ' failed to depict the stripes Jesus took for us.

Not a single inch of Jesus' body was spared from the whipping!

The Stripes of Jesus

Contrary to many popular teachings, it wasn't the crucifixion on the Cross that dealt with our sicknesses and diseases. It was the stripes! In other words, Jesus dealt with all our sicknesses WHEN He took the stripes. And that was prior to His death on the Cross.

1 Peter 2:24 says that Jesus bore our sins in His own body on the tree (Cross). See also Isaiah 53:12. Jesus only dealt with our sins on the Cross (Romans 8:3; Galatians 3:13).

This simply means that **Jesus FIRST paid for our healing before He paid for our remission of sins**. This is a powerful truth!

Therefore, your sins have nothing to do with receiving God's healing for you. Even if your sickness is caused by your own blunder (i.e. STDs or STIs), you are qualified to receive His complete healing!

Disclaimer: I am not advocating anyone to sin. God has called us to bear fruit in keeping with repentance. He desires that we live a holy life.

Every single person whom Jesus healed in the Gospel books was a sinner. They were all living in sin. Their sins were not yet dealt with, because Jesus had yet gone to the Cross! In fact, all of them were healed by 'credit'.

To credit something means that you get to have it before you pay for it. Supposed you enter a cafe and order a cup of latte. The payment is on credit, because you get to enjoy the coffee first, before you call for the bill. The staff needs to place his or her faith in you, trusting that you will make the payment after you enjoy what you have ordered.

Similarly, the people in the Gospel had to place their faith in Jesus, trusting that He would eventually pay for the healing by receiving the stripes. Only by His stripes could they be healed. Their healing was on credit. Jesus had to pay for the healing by taking the stripes, just as He had to pay for the forgiveness He already granted to the people in the Gospel book, by dying on the Cross (Romans 3:23-26).

If Jesus didn't take the stripes, God would be a liar. And all those healings would fail and not be permanent. In addition, **the whole Universe would break apart, because God upholds the Universe by the Word of His power** (Hebrews 1:3; Colossians 1:17).

Healing is significant and essential. It is not a small deal that we can overlook. It is not 'whatever will be, will be.' It speaks of the very nature of God, His integrity and His promise. He does NOT lie (Hebrews 6:18)!

Before Jesus took the stripes, healing was on credit. After Jesus took the stripes, healing was fully paid for us! Let's go back to the cafe analogy. If you first pay for the cup of latte before you have it, the staff doesn't need to place his or her trust in you to make the payment. You already paid for it! In the staff's perspective, the payment is done. It's a reality.

Similarly, when Jesus took the stripes, the payment for healing was done. Completed. It's a reality. You don't have to try harder to put your trust in Him. You can simply receive your healing by the fact that Jesus already paid for it!

The moment you think about the stripes, you can be certain that HEALING IS YOURS!

How Should I Receive My Healing?

The way you receive healing is the same way you receive salvation of your spirit. As I mentioned in Chapter 2, the full meaning of salvation (root word 'sozo') includes healing, deliverance and complete well-being. If you can receive salvation of your spirit by simply believing, then you can receive healing freely by the same token.

Heal the sick, cleanse the lepers, raise the dead, cast out demons. ***Freely*** *you have received, freely give. - Matthew 10:8*

The word 'freely' in Greek means 'a gift that is unearned and undeserved.' It can also mean 'effortlessly'. The context of this passage talks about healing, deliverance and raising of the dead.

In other words, healing is freely given by God. Healing is unearned and undeserved. Healing is **by grace through faith** ----- exactly the same as the salvation of the spirit!

You cannot earn healing. You cannot claim healing based on your own merits or godliness. By trying to earn healing, you disqualify yourself from receiving it. On the other hand, you cannot do anything right to deserve healing. Stop beating yourself up for the mistakes you have done. Stop thinking that you are not good enough to receive healing.

The healing equation has nothing to do with you. **The only reason you can receive healing is because of the stripes of Jesus. Healing is fully paid for. And you can simply receive it effortlessly, by grace through faith!**

You can say something like, *"Jesus, You took the stripes for me. I am not trying to be healed. By Your stripes, I was healed. And I am healed. Sickness, you have no rights to remain in my body. Leave now and never come back. Father, I thank You for Your goodness. I thank You for redemption. I thank You for healing me. Amen."*

Note: There is no method or specific words in this. It's simply about believing and receiving, by grace through faith.

Is The Manifestation of Healing Instantaneous?

Some teach that there are different kinds of healing, such as creative miracles, etc. I like to keep healing simple, because the Gospel is simple. If the Bible doesn't say otherwise, we should refrain from coming out with other extra-biblical stuff.

While 1 Corinthians 12:9 talks about 'gifts' of healing (healing is singular in Greek), the word 'gifts' could mean that there are different types of healing, such as healing of the spine, healing of cancer, healing of fibroid, healing of migraine and the list goes on ----- all these are God's gifts ('charisma' in Greek) because healing is God's gift (charisma).

Jesus healed all who came to Him in the Gospel. Period. He didn't go into the specifics. Neither should we. **In fact, the more general you are, the more the power of God is evident.** It is either you believe that it's simple or you believe that you need to be specific. According to your belief, it will be done (Matthew 9:29).

I have heard of people speaking long prayers and going into the specifics such as '*certain pressure of the tendon, particular angle and degree of the ligament, etc.*' It is not the many words or the specifics that are going to get people healed. **It is the power of God that gets people healed**.

In fact, all the healings which Jesus did were recorded in simple words, "*be healed*"; "*rise up and walk*"; "*be opened*"; "*stretch out your hand*", etc. **Stay simple, stay general and simply trust God**.

Some differentiate different kinds of healing by saying that the Bible recorded 'cure' ('therapeuo' in Greek) and 'heal' ('iaomai' in Greek) on separate occasions when Jesus ministered to the sick. Those who teach this tend to say that 'cure' refers to healing that is progressive, while 'heal' refers to healing that is instantaneous.

I did a study on that and found out that both words are actually interchangeable and used in the Gospel books (Luke 9:42 and Matthew 17:18). Both passages recorded the same incident but one uses 'therapeuo' while the other uses 'iaomai'. Read also Matthew 8:7-8 where both 'therapeuo' and 'iaomai' are used interchangeably in the same passage.

Let's keep healing simple!

Most of Jesus' healings were instantaneous. Therefore, this is what we should expect – an immediate manifestation of healing.

However, there were occasions when Jesus' healings seemed progressive (Matthew 17:18; Matthew 8:13; Matthew 9:22; Luke 17:14;

Mark 8:22-25). While these incidents appeared to be progressive healings, all of Jesus' healings happened within that hour or that day! As we continue to grow in Him, that is the benchmark we can have. I don't know about you, but that is good news to me! It means that there is MORE I can grow unto Him. There is MORE which I can expect to see!

Having said that, Jesus showed us that the manifestation of healing **can sometimes be progressive**. It may take one day or more. It may even take weeks or months. **As long as we continue to believe, we will see the complete manifestation of healing**. I will share more on the position we have in Christ in the next chapter.

*Now in the morning, as they passed by, they saw the fig tree **dried up from the roots**. And Peter, remembering, said to Him, "Rabbi, look! The fig tree which You cursed has withered away."* - Mark 11:20-21

Jesus cursed the fig tree on the day before. He then went into the Temple to drive out those religious people. The next morning, the fig tree dried up from the roots.

Jesus used this illustration to teach His disciples on faith. He said, "*...whatever things you ask when you pray, **believe that you receive them, and you will have them**.*" - Mark 11:24

Jesus cursed the fig tree and nothing seemed to happen visibly on the spot. Nothing instantaneous appeared to take place. However, Jesus knew that it was done because of what He had said (Mark 11:23). The fig tree actually died from its root. It took close to one day before the result could be seen visibly ---- it dried from the root (hidden in the ground) up to the leaves (visible).

Mark 11:24 says, "*Believe that you receive them, and you will have them.*" In other words, you can believe that your healing is done, and that your sickness has dried up from its root, even if you don't see or feel it visibly at the moment. Manifestation will come!

Do not shrink back thinking that healing is not working. Do not try all kinds of other methods as though healing is not working. **By His stripes, you are healed!** Stand firm and believe!

Note: If you are taking medication, continue to do so unless your body tells you otherwise. As shared in Chapter 2, you can continue to depend on Jesus and trust Him for healing while using medication. Your body will know when the complete manifestation of healing has taken place. Your body will know when you can stop the medication.

Every Sickness Is The Same

In our human's perspective, we think that muscle ache is a small problem and it can be healed easily. On the other hand, we think that terminal diseases such as cancer is a big problem and it must be difficult to be healed. The truth is that in heaven's perspective, **every sickness is of the same level.** The chart below will help you to see clearer.

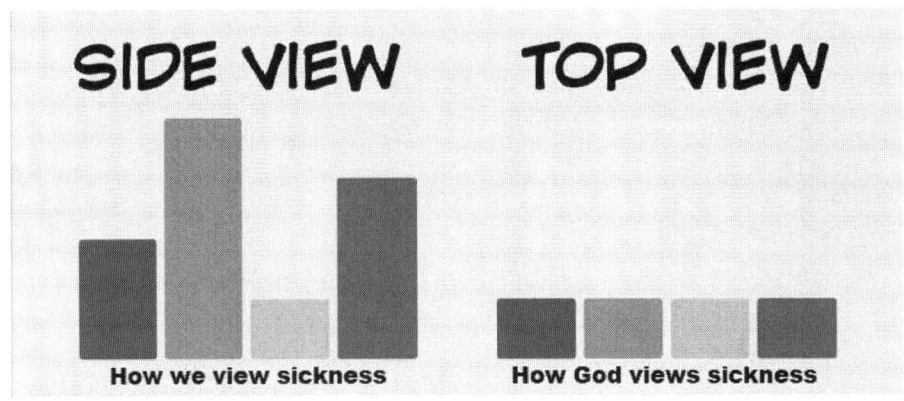

We tend to view sickness from **Side View**, while God views sickness from **Top View**. We think that terminal diseases fall into the 'highest' category, while others like headache and back pain fall into the 'shortest' category. By no means!

Every sickness is in the same category!

Just as God views all kinds of sins as one category ----- sin, God views all kinds of sicknesses and diseases as one category ---- sickness!

If we don't change our perspective on this, we will not see the same result that Jesus saw while He was on earth.

*How God anointed Jesus of Nazareth with the Holy Spirit and with power, who went about doing good and **healing all** who were oppressed by the devil, for God was with Him. - Acts 10:38*

How many did Jesus heal? All! Throughout the Gospel, Jesus didn't spend more time and effort healing the lame and raising the dead as compared to healing someone from a fever. He simply said a few words or laid hands on the sick and they ALL got healed!

*Therefore God also has highly exalted Him and given Him the **name which is above every name**, that at the name of Jesus every knee should bow... - Philippians 2:9-10*

Does sickness have a name? Yes. Cancer is a name. Diabetes is a name. Fibroid is a name. Scoliosis is a name. Tuberculosis is a name. Fever is a name. Every kind of sickness has a name. But the **name of Jesus is the name above every name**. It doesn't matter what kind of sickness you have, because **every sickness must bow at the name of Jesus!**

Whether it is a back problem or cancer, Jesus took the stripes for them all. Jesus' body was required to be flogged and broken for the healing of muscle ache, just as His body was required to be flogged and broken for the healing of cancer. To deem that one sickness is smaller than the other is to make light of what Jesus went through.

He fully paid for our healing. The power of God is either ALL or none.

If you bought a small but expensive pen at $5,000, but you left it in the store; when you reach home, you realize that you have forgotten to take it. What would you do? You will go back to the store and take it, because you have paid for it.

If you bought a large LED TV at $5,000, but you left it in the store; when you reach home, you realize that you have forgotten to take it. What would you do? You will do the same thing as you did to the pen. You will go back and take it. Why? Because you have paid for it.

Jesus paid the same price for every sickness --- whether it is 'small' or 'big' in your eyes. You can take it. To believe and receive healing is to honor what Jesus has paid with His blood. You can confidently take it because the payment is done.

Many exalt the healing testimonies of terminal diseases and 'trivialize' the healing of 'smaller' ones such as backache. They tend to only share 'big' testimonies of healings but seldom talk about the 'small' testimonies of healings. The responses from many also reveal that we are more thankful for the 'big' healings than the 'small' healings. We exclaim, "*Hallelujah! Praise God! That's awesome!*" when someone is healed from cancer. But we go, "*Oh well... that's good*" when someone is healed from headache. We forget that it took Jesus the same sacrifice for both such healings!

God spoke to me one day when I asked Him why we don't see the healing of terminal diseases as easily as the healing of small ailments like headaches and muscle aches. He replied, "**If you can have the same attitude of thanksgiving for the healing of muscle aches just as the healing of terminal diseases, you will see the healing of terminal diseases as easily as the healing of muscle ache.**"

Following this revelation from God, we went to minister to a cancer patient. We prepared him, saying, "*I am not going to pray a long prayer. Just a few simple words. Because it's the stripes of Jesus that you are healed.*" We laid our hand on him and said, "*Be healed.*" That's it. On the following week, he went back for a medical review and was declared cancer-free!

I believe it's all about seeing every kind of sickness from heaven's perspective.

Healing is simple. Don't make it complicated. Don't focus on your sickness and symptoms. **Focus on the truth that Jesus took the stripes so that you can be healed.** Healing is by grace through faith. Healing is yours!

Act As Though You Are Whole

Once you have believed that by His stripes you are healed, you can start speaking and acting as though you are whole.

This is not something psychological. Neither has it to do with the law of attraction or placebo effect.

It is actually biblical.

*Therefore I tell you, whatever you ask in prayer, **believe that you have received it**, and it will be yours.* - Mark 11:24

How do you show that you believe that you have received it? **You act as though you have received it**.

I give you an illustration. Imagine your father says, "*I have sent $50,000 into your bank account.*" You haven't managed to check that account. But you respond, "Thank you!" You believe that you have received the amount.

How do you show that you believe it? You go ahead and buy something you wanted to get. **By acting on it, you actually show that you believe** that you have received the money.

This is the same for healing. You have believed -------- '*By His stripes, you are healed.*' You have received it. Now you act into it. **Your action follows.**

If a thing is in the Bible, it is so; it is not even to be prayed about; it is to be received and acted upon. - Smith Wigglesworth, on the Power of the Word of God.

The man with the withered hand acted upon it and **<u>stretched out</u>** his hand (Matthew 12:13).

The man with the infirmity of 38 years acted upon it, took his bed and **<u>walked</u>** (John 5:9).

The lame man acted upon it, **<u>leaped up</u>**, stood and walked (Acts 3:8).

The paralytic acted upon it, **got up**, picked up his bed and walked (Mark 2:12).

*"It is a law of the human mind that **I can act myself into believing faster** than I can believe myself into acting."* - John G Lake, the late American healing evangelist (1870-1935)

Chapter 4:

The Great Position

Healing Is The Position You Stand On

Chapter 1 of this manual establishes the foundation of your position in Christ. Christ has redeemed us from every sickness and disease. You were not created to fall sick and die. Stop saying like the world says, "*Everybody will grow old, fall sick and die.*" You are in the world but not of the world.

You are meant to walk in health and live an abundant life (John 10:10).

You are not the sick trying to be healed. You are the healed resisting sickness. Healing is a position we already have in Christ, not a condition we are going to have.

Even if you are having a physical condition right now, your condition is not your conclusion. Your position is. **Stay in your position and it will conclude your condition ----- wholeness!**

Whatever Christ has done for you is your position. Nothing can ever change that. By His stripes, you were healed. Positionally, you are already healed. **In God's perspective, you are healed.** What is left for you to experience is the manifestation of that healing.

Positional: You Are Healed!

Experiential: Manifestation of the healing.

What lies between the positional and the experiential is **mind renewal**.

*And do not be conformed to this world, but be transformed by the renewing of your mind, **that you may prove** what is that good and acceptable and perfect will of God. - Romans 12:2*

To be able to prove that something actually works shows that it already did.

Healing is '*that good and acceptable and perfect will of God*.' When our mind is renewed, we will experience the positional.

The Battle Of The Mind

The enemy is a master in the carnal realm of our mind. If we choose to fight him from that realm, we are bound to lose. He is a liar (John 8:44) and his job is to plant thoughts that sound like you or even like God into your mind, so that you will believe his lie and eat its fruit.

*For the weapons of our warfare are **not carnal** but mighty in God for pulling down strongholds, casting down arguments and every high thing that **exalts itself against the knowledge of God**, bringing every thought into captivity to the obedience of Christ.* - 2 Corinthians 10:4-5

Spiritual warfare is not so much about binding territorial spirits or doing a prayer walk. In fact, you don't see Jesus and the disciples (including apostle Paul) doing any of these. The whole of the New Testament epistles contains truths for the renewing of your mind (Romans 12:2). Why? Because spiritual warfare mostly has to do with your mind. That is the real place of battle. The devil will fight you there. He is very subtle because he is like a thief who steals, kills and destroys (John 10:10). More often than not, he wants to steal the truth from you about your identity and your inheritance as sons and daughters of God. This is why we need to establish ourselves in the Redemption of Christ ------- what He did for us on the Cross and who He made us to be, so that we can train our senses to discern between good and evil (Hebrews 5:13-14).

69

"Healing is not really working, is it?"

"If God wants to heal you, He would have already done it."

"So and so also died of the same sickness. He was a man of God, you know?"

"You are going to die. What's the point?"

"Are you sure you can be healed?"

"Maybe it's not God's timing yet."

"Something is wrong with you. That's the reason why God didn't heal you."

"Are you sure you have been healed? You feel the pain and the symptoms now. You probably weren't healed then."

The above are simply some subtle lies that the enemy speaks into your mind. This is the time you should not react to them. You don't want to entertain the enemy or converse with him. You want to stay in communion with God and focus on Him. Each time when a lie enters your mind, you take that opportunity to establish truths in communion with God.

Note: You can only establish truths in communion with God if you know the Word. This is why it is so vital to interpret who God is based on who Jesus is in the Scriptures!

Let me give you an example. Supposed someone sitting beside you has a bad cough. The thought may come, *"This cough is really bad and it's contagious, you know?"* This thought obviously sounded like your own voice, but it's the enemy planting it into your mind, inducing fear so that you would believe and receive the sickness.

If you are having that thought coming in, grab this opportunity to commune with God. You can respond, *"Father, I thank You for Redemption. Christ has redeemed me from every sickness. I thank You for divine protection in Psalm 91 ---- that a thousand may fall on my side, and ten thousand on my right hand, but none shall come near me. Not even this flu. I thank You for Your love and Your goodness. Thank You for giving me life and life in abundance."*

You are crushing the lie with truth and you are taking the chance to develop intimacy with God through communion. What an extreme privilege you and I have! The enemy might think that he could pull you away from God with his lies, but little does he realize that he is actually pushing you to go deeper with God!

God has given you and me the mind of Christ (1 Corinthians 2:16). However, you can still choose to function from the carnal mind (Romans 8:5-7). The carnal mind is always hostile against God. In other words, it will always contradict the truth, often in a subtle way. If we function in the carnal mind, it produces death (Romans 8:6) ----- death in every form, and in the context of this manual, sickness.

*For the weapons of our warfare are **not carnal** but mighty in God for pulling down strongholds, casting down arguments and every high thing that **exalts itself against the knowledge of God**, bringing every thought into captivity to the obedience of Christ.* - 2 Corinthians 10:4-5

How do you pull down strongholds? It says 'casting down arguments and every high thing that exalts itself against the knowledge of God.' When we function with our carnal mind, we exalt itself against the knowledge of God. Because the carnal mind is always hostile against God. This is why it says that the weapons of our warfare are not carnal. So how do you pull down strongholds? We need to bring every thought into captivity to the obedience of Christ. In other words, we need to subject it to the mind of Christ. If it's not what the mind of Christ is saying, then ignore it. Those are lies. People are held in bondage and sickness because of these lies that they believe in.

The doctor may say, "*You are going to die. Cancer has spread to your organs.*" That's the carnal mind speaking. But what does the mind of Christ say? "*By His stripes, I am healed. He Himself took my infirmities and bore my diseases.*" You declare, "*Cancer, you have to go right now in Jesus' name!*"

We have the mind of Christ. We need to renew our mind. **Renewing our mind is simply about functioning in the mind of Christ and agreeing with what God says**. It's about shifting from the old mindset to the new mindset in every area of our lives ------ in this context, healing.

You are a new creation. Your old man (nature) had died. Your old mind had died. Now you are a new man. You have the mind of Christ. You are not trying to work on your old mind. It is already dead (Romans 6:6). You are learning to operate with your new mind.

Functioning in the mind of Christ is about setting our minds on the things of the Spirit. Since the enemy 'battles' you in the carnal realm, you cannot overcome him in that realm. It produces death (Romans 8:6). Instead, you need to think and move in the realm of the Spirit ------- that is where life is! **To function in the realm of the Spirit is to simply believe in the Word** (John 6:63).

For example, the carnal mind says that it is normal to be down with common flu. **Common flu may be common to men, but it is not common to you because you are not a common man**. You are uncommon, holy and set apart. Christ has redeemed you from sickness to walk and live in health!

Which part of the Bible says that when you are old, you will have sickness? Which part of the Scriptures says that when you are old, you will have weak knees and aching joints? That's what the world says, not what the Word says. We need to renew our mind.

Moses died at 120. His eyes were undimmed and his strength did not leave him (Deuteronomy 34:7). Caleb, at the age of 85, was as strong as when he was 40 (Joshua 14:10-11). And they were all living in the Old Covenant. We have a more superior Covenant than them! They didn't have the Spirit of Christ living in them. We have!

There are some crazy, personal testimonies that I can't share here in this manual. There is some stuff that I do personally at the expense of my life, because I have to walk out this message that I preach on divine healing and health. I'm not including it in this manual, because I am concerned that some are not ready for it and may find it ridiculous or even take unnecessary offense, causing them to be unable to receive the main purpose of this manual, which is divine healing! It may also backfire or cause some to follow blindly without proper understanding. **My heart is really for you and your loved ones to be healed.**

What I can say is that as believers, we are not meant to go from healing to healing. **We are meant to go from healing to divine health ------ never sick again**! This statement shouldn't make anyone feel condemned or 'smaller'. It is a privilege that we can all grow into. It means that there is **MORE** in this journey as a Christian. I want to grow unto everything that Jesus is ------ love, character, the heart for the lost and **ALSO health!**

If we talk about the need to walk in love as He does, then we also need to walk in health like He does. We cannot pick and choose which area we want to be like Christ. It is either ALL or none. He said, "*Follow Me.*" He has sacrificed His life to make it possible and accessible for us to follow Him in every area. This is the grace of God. What a great Abba Father we have! Let's focus on knowing Him and keep growing!

Note: If you get 'hit' by the enemy with sickness, the devil doesn't know that he is actually sending you into the training ground to go deeper in seeing the goodness of God! I believe that we can walk in a place completely free from the hit of the enemy (Ephesians 6:16; Psalm 91).

Divine Health As Believers In Christ

While the stripes of Jesus paid for our healing, the Cross of Jesus paid for our health. On the Cross, Jesus redeemed us from the curse of sicknesses and diseases (Galatians 3:13) to walk in divine health.

Jesus Himself is our example. He walked in divine health throughout His life on earth in the Gospel books. There was not a single record of Him needing healing. This is not interpreting from omission. This is because He had no sin and did no sin (1 John 3:5; 2 Corinthians 5:21; 1 Peter 2:22). Since every form of death only came as a result of sin (Romans 5:21), Jesus had no form of death (which includes sickness) because He was sinless. He could give life because He IS LIFE (John 14:6; Romans 5:17; 1 Corinthians 15:45).

The stripes couldn't kill Him. The nails couldn't kill Him. The crucifixion couldn't kill Him. He couldn't die because death couldn't reign in Him who had no sin. Therefore, He had to be hung on the Cross (Galatians 3:13) so that He could become sin (2 Corinthians 5:21) and took the curse and death that we deserved. He gave up His life on His own (John 10:17-18; Luke 23:46; John 19:30).

The Bible says in 1 John 4:17 that '*As He is, so are we in this world.*' We are often taught that whatever Jesus is right now in heaven, we are the same in this world. Since Jesus is healthy, we are healthy in this world. While the principle is true, the context of this passage is actually talking about the love that has been perfected by Christ, so that we can have the boldness to face God in the Day of Judgment, because we have been made righteous in Christ (through His love), as Christ is before the Father.

Having said that, we have been given the Spirit of Christ to be like Him (Ephesians 2:6; Colossians 3:1; 1 Corinthians 1:30; 2 Corinthians 13:5) ------- that includes walking in divine health on earth like Jesus!

Jesus taught His disciples to pray in Matthew 6:10, "*Your kingdom come. Your will be done, **on earth as it is in heaven**.*"

It is in God's heart and His will that the earth reflects what is in heaven. Heaven has no sickness. Therefore, sickness cannot be in you on earth.

Critics will point out certain passages about the apostle Paul, Timothy, Epaphroditus and Trophimus. Let's take a quick look at these.

Apostle Paul's So-Called Infirmity

*And lest I should be exalted above measure by the abundance of the revelations, a **thorn in the flesh** was given to me, a messenger of satan to buffet me, lest I be exalted above measure. Concerning this thing I pleaded with the Lord three times that it might depart from me. And He said to me, "**My grace is sufficient for you, for My strength is made perfect in weakness.**" Therefore most gladly I will rather boast in my **infirmities**, that the power of Christ may rest upon me.* - 2 Corinthians 12:7-9

Many used this passage to say that Paul's thorn in the flesh was a physical infirmity. They based it on verse 9 - "*....I will rather boast in my infirmities...*" There are others who say that Paul had eye disease (Galatians 4:13-15; Galatians 6:11).

We need to read Scriptures in context. Paul said that the thorn in the flesh was given by a messenger of satan (not God) to prevent him from being exalted because of surpassing revelations He received from God. God cannot be giving anyone sickness as Jesus is the will of God clearly revealed, and He went about healing all who were sick.

As we look deeper, we will realize that Paul didn't receive this thorn in the flesh because he was prideful. In fact, he was stopped by satan from being exalted (lifted up) with a greater influence so that he couldn't go on and impact even more lives for Jesus!

The thorn in the flesh was first mentioned in Numbers 33. We can apply the Law of First Mention into the Scriptures if it is not explicitly explained.

But if you do not drive out the inhabitants of the land from before you, then it shall be that those whom you let remain shall be irritants in your eyes and **thorns in your sides***, and they shall harass you in the land where you dwell.* - Numbers 33:55

The phrase 'thorns in your sides' is synonymous with the phrase 'thorn in the flesh'. Over here, it speaks of the enemies who would continually harass God's people. Sounds familiar?

Throughout apostle Paul's ministry, he was always persecuted by the religious Jews (Acts 13:45; 14:19; Acts 23:12). In fact, he faced persecutions by the enemies of God (the religious Jews and others) throughout his ministry.

And see, now I go bound in the spirit to Jerusalem, not knowing the things that will happen to me there, except that the Holy Spirit testifies in every city, saying that **chains and tribulations await me***.* - Acts 20:22-23

The phrase '**thorn in the flesh**' is actually **the persecution he faced by the religious ones**. This is why even though he prayed to God to remove it, God did not remove but said, "*My grace is sufficient for you...*" Because God has promised persecution to believers who want to live godly (2 Timothy 3:12). If it were sickness, God cannot and will not reply the same way, because He is Jehovah Rapha (Exodus 15:26)!

The word 'infirmities' in 2 Corinthians 12:9 is 'astheneia' (in Greek), which can be translated as 'weakness.' It is the exact same word used in this verse, *"My grace is sufficient for you, for My strength is made perfect in* **weakness***."*

Paul boasted in his weakness in a chapter before this.

With far greater labors, far more imprisonments, with countless beatings, and often near death. Five times I received at the hands of the Jews the forty lashes less one. Three times I was beaten with rods. Once I was stoned. Three times I was shipwrecked; a night and a day I was adrift at sea; on frequent journeys, in danger from rivers, danger from robbers, danger from my own people, danger from Gentiles, danger in the city, danger in the wilderness, danger at sea, danger from false brothers; in toil and hardship, through many a sleepless night, in hunger and thirst, often without food, in cold and exposure. And, apart from other things, there is the daily pressure on me of my anxiety for all the churches. **Who is weak, and I am not weak**? *Who is made to fall, and I am not indignant? If I must boast,* **I will boast of the things that show my weakness**. - 2 Corinthians 11:23-30

The word 'weakness' in this passage is the exact same word 'astheneia', used in 2 Corinthians 12:9. Paul recounted his infirmities (or weaknesses), and sickness was NOT on the list!

Why then did Paul talk about his physical infirmity in Galatians 4:13-15?

Firstly, the word 'infirmity' is the same word ('astheneia') used for weakness. Secondly, before Paul preached to the Galatians, he was stoned and had a near-death experience (Acts 14:19-22)! By the way, our understanding of stoning may be very different in the 21st century. In those days, stoning was the capital punishment of the Jews. The congregation would use rocks to stone the person until he is dead.

Right after Paul was stoned until he almost died (the Jews thought he died), he went to preach in Derbe on the following day! Derbe, Lystra, Iconium and Antioch were all cities in the region of Galatia (Acts 14:20-21). Hence, it wouldn't be surprising for Paul to be bodily weak, preaching to the Galatians right after experiencing the stoning and persecution from the Jews.

*You know that because of **physical infirmity** I preached the gospel to you at the first.* - Galatians 4:13

Since we have established earlier that we should let the explicit (clear) interpret the implicit (unclear), Paul's infirmity couldn't be sickness. Rather, it was a physical weakness due to severe persecution (stoning).

Timothy's So-Called Stomach Ailment

The critics and skeptics often use 1 Timothy 5:23 to prove against divine healing.

No longer drink only water, but use a little wine for your stomach's sake and your frequent infirmities. - 1 Timothy 5:23

Before we are quick to jump into the conclusion that Paul didn't manage to heal Timothy, we need to understand that in those days, water was often contaminated. Contaminated water caused stomach issues.

Paul, in his wisdom, obviously recognized the cause of Timothy's stomach problem. The latter kept drinking contaminated water. To prevent this from happening, Paul suggested that Timothy should use a little wine. The word 'use' in Greek means to 'employ' or to 'make use of'. In other words, Paul was saying, "*Stop drinking only water.*

Employ/make use of a little wine. Mix it with water." The ancient Greeks and Romans often drank their water mixed with wine to purify and kill the bacteria in the contaminated water.

If we supposed that Paul really didn't manage to heal Timothy (assumed by the critics), which cannot be proven in Scriptures, we need to know that the ultimate model we are to follow isn't Paul. It's Jesus.

When it comes to loving people, we are on the same page -------- "*We must love others as Jesus loves.*" But when it comes to healing, we suddenly change our mind, "*We must follow Paul instead of Jesus.*" Is that even biblical? If Jesus is our ultimate model for love, then He must be our ultimate model for healing and health. If we want to model after Jesus in love, then let us also model after Him in power.

Epaphroditus Was Sick Almost Unto Death

*For indeed he was **sick** almost unto death; but God had mercy on him, and not only on him but on me also, lest I should have sorrow upon sorrow.* - Philippians 2:27

Some claim that Paul didn't manage to heal his fellow minister, Epaphroditus. The word 'sick' is 'astheneo' in Greek, which can be translated as 'sick' or 'weak'. The following verses reveal what actually happened to Epaphroditus.

*Receive him therefore in the Lord with all gladness, and hold such men in esteem; because **for the work of Christ he came close to death**, not regarding his life...* - Philippians 2:29-30

Epaphroditus almost died because of the work of Christ. He could have been beaten up, stoned or simply exhausted ------ resulting in weakness. We are not sure as it is not recorded in the Scriptures.

The good news is this ------------ he was healed (Philippians 2:27-28)!

Trophimus Left Sick By Paul

*Erastus stayed in Corinth, but Trophimus I have left in Miletus **sick**.* - 2 Timothy 4:20

The word 'sick' here is translated either as 'weak' or 'sick'. We don't know if Trophimus was really sick or he was simply worn out (fatigue) traveling and laboring with Paul. Paul's ministry was extremely difficult (2 Corinthians 11:23-27; Colossians 1:29). Ministering with him would have been pretty exhausting.

Paul could have left Trophimus to rest, while he continued to advance the Gospel.

IMPORTANT: We cannot use one unclear verse to build a theology around it. Instead, we can be certain of God's will for healing and health through many passages in the Scriptures, especially in the person and life of Jesus.

Remember: Apostle Paul himself said that he was still growing in knowing Christ and the power of His resurrection (Philippians 3:10-12). Even if we assume that Paul didn't manage to heal one of these people whom we talked about, he isn't the ultimate example. Jesus is!

Establishing Your Position

Do not be complacent with your position. Do not think that once you understood the truth, it would always stay there permanently. Sometimes, it is good to remind ourselves and **stay established in the truth** (2 Peter 1:12). We live in the world and it is still possible for the world's perspective to get into our mind (John 13:10; Romans 12:2). What you read and receive can affect you. I usually avoid using Google to search about symptoms of any sickness. The more you research about the symptoms, the more you will be convinced negatively about the implications. What produces in you often becomes fear, instead of faith. Faith comes by hearing and hearing from the Word of God (Romans 10:17). Instead of feeding yourself with news and articles, feed yourself with the Word of God. The Word is the truth!

This is a prayer that I often pray ------ when I feel the need to establish myself in the truth in communion with God. As I shared before, it is not a method. It's about relationship and communion. Method doesn't work. The problem is when we turn what works into a formula or method. Relationship and communion are the key ------- because it speaks of trust.

"Father, I thank You for the Body and the Blood of Jesus. I appreciate Your love and Your goodness for me. Jesus, You died for me. And You paid for me to walk in healing and health. I thank You for Your Body, broken for me. Your Body was broken so that mine can be whole. Your Body was bruised so that mine is well. Your bones were exposed so that mine never ever has to be exposed. I thank You that Your Body removed sin from me, and along with sin, Your Body removed every effect and every curse of sin ----- which includes every

82

sickness, disease, pain, injury, accident, premature death, tiredness and exhaustion. Jesus, I thank You that while Your Body removed sin from me, Your Blood removed me from sin. Your Blood remitted and sent away all my sins. Your Blood redeemed me to the beginning before the Fall. It is as though I had never partaken in the fruit of the tree of knowledge of good and evil. Father, You look at me, as though I have never sinned before. You look at me, as if You are looking at Your Son Jesus ---- righteous, holy, blameless and perfect in Your sight. And if I have never sinned before, I can never suffer any effect and consequence of sin. Who Christ is, I am. What He has, I have. Therefore, I thank You that I have divine life living within me. The Spirit that raised Christ from the dead lives in me. The Spirit that heals every sickness and disease lives in me. I thank You that I have divine health, protection, wholeness, peace and joy. Thank You Jesus! I thank You for Your love for me. I rest in Your goodness and faithfulness. I rest in You. Amen."

I can't tell how many times the onset of mild flu symptoms (discomfort of the throat) left me completely by simply establishing myself in the truth.

If You Know Your Identity, Health Is Your Reality

Your identity as a son/daughter of God gives you access to divine health (Galatians 3:26; Galatians 4:6; Romans 8:11).

The enemy will try his best to hit you off your identity ground. It has been his tactic since day one (Genesis 3:5). He caused Man to doubt his identity ------ Adam was already created to be like God (Genesis 1:26-27).

Today, the enemy wants us to doubt our identity so that we will continually strive to become someone else, instead of already being the sons and the daughters that Jesus has paid a high price for! Identity is so important (it is everything!) but it is a huge topic. Since we are focused on healing, we will only touch on the aspect that covers healing and health.

The enemy will want to knock you off your identity ground for healing and health. He will be relentless. This is why we need to stand firm and keep our armor on.

*Put on the **whole armor of God**, that you may be able to **stand against the wiles of the devil**. For we do not wrestle against flesh and blood, but against principalities, against powers, against the rulers of the darkness of this age, against spiritual hosts of wickedness in the heavenly places. Therefore **take up the whole armor of God**, that you may be able to **withstand in the evil day, and having done all, to stand**.* - Ephesians 6:11-13

We have to know that our fight is not physical. It is spiritual. It is a war between two kingdoms: The Kingdom of God VS the kingdom of darkness.

While we advance the kingdom of God, there is another kingdom that wars against us to prevent the kingdom from advancing. **The fight is never personal or physical. The fight is always about the kingdom.** The enemy is not against you, because if God is for you, who can be against you? The enemy is against the One in you. You have died and now Christ lives in and through you (Galatians 2:20). The enemy is against the kingdom within you. **If he can stop you, he can stop the kingdom from advancing.** He doesn't want you to know that healing is simple. He doesn't want you to experience the manifestation of healing. Because once you have tasted it, he knows that he can NEVER stop you from reaching the lost and healing the sick!

However, if we take this war as something personal, we will not be able to stand and endure. We end up in self-pity and self-focused. We end up doubting who God is and who we are. That disarms our kingdom armor and allows the enemy to steal, kill and destroy.

If we know that this war is against the kingdom of God, we will be kingdom-focused and Christ-focused. Our kingdom armor becomes the shield of faith we can take to extinguish all the flaming arrows of the evil one (Ephesians 6:16).

With this in mind, we are ready to stand our ground and remain immovable.

The armor of God is like our identity which comprises of truth, righteousness, peace, faith, salvation, Word and Spirit (Ephesians 6:14-18). If you notice, experience is never on the list. Experiences are real but they may not be the truth. We must never allow experiences to define our identity. Don't let what you are going through define your identity. Don't let your reality define your identity. **Always let what Christ has gone through define your identity.**

Stand Firm In Your Identity

Whether you have experienced partial healing or are still experiencing the symptoms of the sickness, you need to stand firm on your identity ground.

*...and having done all, **to stand**.* - Ephesians 6:13

Even if you are still feeling the pain; you continue to stand firm in the truth that by His stripes, you were healed. Stay in that place. Camp there. Live there. **DO NOT BE MOVED**. Eventually, your experience will catch up with the truth. **The manifestation will surely come.**

"I am not moved by what I see. I am moved only by what I believe." - Smith Wigglesworth, the late British faith healer (1859-1947)

You can pray something like, *"Father, I thank You that I am not trying to be healed. By the stripes of Jesus, I was healed and I am healed. I remain healed. Therefore, sickness and symptoms, you have no right to remain in my body. You have nothing against me. You have no hold in me. In Jesus' name, I command you to leave right now! Get out and never return again! Body, I command you to be completely whole now! Father, I thank You for Your goodness. I rest and trust in Your faithfulness, goodness and health. I thank You for redemption."*

Note: I have to reiterate that this is not a method for you to pray. It's about having communion with God and believing in Him.

Even after you have experienced wholeness, you still need to stand firm in your identity. Because the enemy will still try to 'steal' your healing. He will plant thoughts into your mind, bringing familiar symptoms and pain in your body, and causing you to think that you are not really healed.

Let me share something that will help you.

A few years ago, when I was in the Gents, a sudden thought came to my mind. I had a flashback of how I had difficulty getting up from bed in the past, due to the autoimmune disease. After that flashback, I found myself having difficulty getting up from the toilet bowl. There was a sharp pain at the back of my pelvis. It was a very familiar symptom of the autoimmune disease. Then a thought came, "*Maybe I am not healed fully after all.*"

Remember, the voice of the enemy sounds exactly like yours.

Instead of entertaining that thought, I immediately turned to God in communion, "*Father, I thank You that I have been healed and I remain healed. Symptom and pain, you have no right to be here. Jesus, You are so good to me. I thank You for Your complete and perfect work on the Cross. I thank You for Your stripes.*"

Immediately, the sharp pain disappeared! I walked out of the Gents, leaping with joy. This incident reaffirmed the importance of knowing our position and identity.

The enemy will try to put lying symptoms in your body. He wants you to doubt your healing and believe in his lies. If you believe him, you will receive the sickness back into your body. Don't waste time trying to fight him. Take the opportunity to commune with God and worship Him.

Therefore **submit to God**. *Resist the devil and he will flee from you.* - James 4:7

Believe Only In The Word, Not The World

If you believe in what the world says, the world will define your world. But if you **believe in what the Word says, the Word will define your world.**

In today's world, researches on medical health have been changing. Sometimes, they even contradict one another. One research can say that certain food and drinks are bad for your health, while another will say that the same food and drinks are good for your health. Instead of being swayed to the left and right by going after the researches, go after the Word of God. For it is the only unchanging truth.

Medical doctors may say that your sickness has gone into remission. In their perspective, it means that your sickness is now inactive, and there is a possible chance for relapse. But you need to turn the word 'remission' from the world's perspective to God's perspective. The word 'remission' in Greek is 'aphesis', which means 'something sent away'. This was first illustrated in Leviticus 16 as the Azazel goat (or the goat of departure) on the Day of Atonement. It was the scapegoat that took the sins of Israel and then was sent away into the wilderness. Jesus, on the day of Redemption, became our scapegoat and took all our sins. Because of His sacrifice, our sins were fully remitted (Hebrews 9:15, 22) and we have been redeemed. Biblical remission, therefore, speaks of complete freedom. You can say, "*Father, I thank You for the redemption of Christ. I thank You that my sickness has gone into remission. It is sent away. It is removed. It will never return again. I thank You that I have complete freedom. I am completely healed.*"

Note: Every prayer example I gave in this manual is not a method of prayer. It is just an example of communion. Many like to confess the words of prayer, thinking that it will work. It won't. Confession alone doesn't get you anything. Believing does. Yes, there is a place for confession. If you believe, you will speak it out. If you don't believe, speak until you believe. Change your words and it will eventually change your mind and your belief. Ultimately, it is the 'believing' that brings the 'receiving'.

Sometimes, we can be very religious. We pray the right prayers. But the words that we say (as a lifestyle) outside of our prayer contradict the prayers we pray. We can pray, "*Jesus, I thank You that by Your stripes, I am healed. I am not trying to be healed. I am healed. I am the healed resisting sickness.*"

Then a friend or colleague sees us experiencing pain or symptoms in the body. He asks, "*How are you?*" And we respond, "*Still in pain*" or "*Not doing good*". When a church mate asks, "*How are you?*" We respond, "*Not healed yet.*" The words we say **outside of our prayer reveal our belief** more than the prayer we pray.

We can actually respond, "*I'm relying on God each day*" or "*I'm recovering; I'm getting better through Him.*" This is not lying. You are speaking in alignment with the Word ----- that is the truth! You can choose to be diplomatically correct and die early. Or you can choose to be biblically correct, be laughed at and live long (Psalm 91:16). Jesus was laughed at when He told the people that the girl was not dead but sleeping (Luke 8:52; Matthew 9:24). In reality, she was dead. But in God's perspective, she was sleeping, because she would be raised from the dead.

Believing is not denying our reality. Believing is denying our reality its power, **with the power and truth of God's Word**.

Minister Healing To Someone

Praise God when you experience healing completely (or instantly) by reading this manual and meditating on His Word.

However, should the manifestation of healing not be completed yet, start ministering healing to others as you continue to trust Him for complete wholeness. In the next chapter, I will share how you can heal the sick.

I know this opposes your flesh. You don't feel like doing it. But we are not called to live by feelings. We are called to live by faith.

The enemy will try his best to stop you. He'll say, "*Come on... you are not healed. How can you heal others? Please, get yourself healed first.*"

"*What if someone sees that I have a physical condition? It's embarrassing to minister healing to him.*"

"*Physician! Heal yourself!*"

"*Who am I to minister healing when I am still struggling?*"

"*Where is my credibility?*"

"*I am not whole yet. Why should I help others?*"

"*I am still in pain. People will reject me when I approach them, because I'm a bad testimony.*"

This list goes on. Let me crush that once and for all ------ these are the voices of the enemy. His goal is to stop you from ministering healing to others. He is fearful of that. He is afraid that you receive your healing and that others receive theirs and acknowledge Jesus as their Lord!

There were a number of times in the past when I persisted to minister healing to others in the streets when I was still in pain. After ministering healing to them, my pain suddenly disappeared.

Some teach that this is sowing and reaping. You sow healing; you reap healing. However, I don't see this kind of sowing and reaping in the New Covenant. In fact, because of what Jesus did, we can now reap what we did not sow (John 4:37-38; Isaiah 53:4-5). Jesus reaped what we sowed, so that we can reap what He sowed. We sowed disobedience, sin, etc. Jesus reaped these on the Cross. Jesus sowed obedience, righteousness, etc. And we reaped them because of the Cross!

By ministering healing to others when you are still trusting God for complete manifestation of healing, it actually reinforces your belief ------ that you believe that it's God's will and desire for you to be whole.

Before we proceed to the next chapter, Chapter 1 to 4 are more than enough for you to receive your healing as the foundations have been laid. Go back and read all over again. Take time to meditate on the Scriptures. Commune with Him. Let the Spirit of Life within you imparts wholeness to your body.

*Healing is not by striving or **wresting**. It is by **RESTING** in the perfect love and goodness of God through Jesus' finished works.*

*Healing is not by **doing** more. It is by knowing that it has been **DONE**.*

*Healing is not by **trying** harder. It is by **TRUSTING**.*

*Healing is not by **achieving**. It is by **RECEIVING**.*

As I shared at the beginning before Chapter 1, the purpose of this manual is to renew your mind so that you can believe Jesus and receive your healing and health. You can't really believe in your heart if the stronghold of lies is not replaced by truths. This manual destroys lies and half-truths (which are still lies) and imparts truths into you so that you can believe right and be set free (John 8:32).

Remember: Healing is SIMPLE ------ ONLY believe (Mark 5:36) **and SIMPLY believe** (Mark 9:23)!

Take some time right NOW to meditate on His body and His blood. Don't rush through this communion. Thank Him for His stripes. Thank Him for the Cross. Thank Him for the Spirit of Life whom He has given to you. The presence of Divine Life is within you. Allow that Life to permeate every part of your body, crushing every symptom, sickness and disease. Thank Him that by His stripes, you are healed. Stay in that place of communion.

Chapter 5:
The Great Ministry

Apart from the four-fold offices (Ephesians 4:11), believers only have one ministry recorded in the Bible.

*Now all things are of God, who has reconciled us to Himself through Jesus Christ, and has given us **the ministry of reconciliation**.* - 2 Corinthians 5:18

Jesus didn't have a healing ministry. Neither should you and I have one. The reason why we are called to heal the sick is to reconcile men and women back to their heavenly Father. Healing reveals the heart of God to the lost so that they want to return to His loving arms.

Note: In the Greek, pastors and teachers are classified under one office. This is why I mentioned four-fold offices. A pastor must be able to teach. Else he cannot shepherd his flocks.

Your Qualification

Mark 16:17-18 says that believers shall lay hands on the sick. It wasn't a request from Jesus. **It was a command.** Jesus told His disciples to heal the sick (Matthew 10:8).

Firstly, we need to establish the truth that every believer is qualified to heal the sick.

He who believes *and is baptized will be saved; but he who does not believe will be condemned. And **these signs will follow those who believe***: *In My name they will cast out demons; they will speak with new tongues; they will take up serpents; and if they drink anything deadly, it will by no means hurt them; **they will lay hands on the sick, and they will recover***. - Mark 16:16-18

It says, "These signs follow those who believe..." It doesn't say, "These signs follow the healing evangelists, the pastors, the leaders, the holy ones, the fasted ones, the mature believers, the sinless ones, etc."

If you read the passage in context, Jesus was talking about NEW believers who would be saved! **You can be born again one minute ago and be healing the sick the very next minute!** As long as you believe in Christ, these signs WILL follow you. In other words, you don't even have to pursue signs and wonders. As a believer, signs and wonders pursue you!

In fact, it is often easier to see the new believers healing the sick than the 'older' believers, because the latter has believed many sacred cows throughout their Christian journey.

Don't disqualify what Jesus has already qualified.

How Did Jesus Qualify Us?

The first Adam was a created man. But the second and the last Adam came to show us how a redeemed Man looked like. Jesus needed to be anointed by the Holy Spirit (Acts 10:38) to provide us with the example of how a redeemed Man could walk in the fullness of God -------- both power and love. You and I are now the redeemed men and women of God.

Jesus Himself fulfilled all righteousness after He was baptized in water (Matthew 3:15). Then heaven was torn open (Mark 1:10) and the fullness of God's blessings (Deuteronomy 28) came upon Jesus -------- the Spirit of God. The Father said, "*This is My Beloved Son, in whom I am well-pleased.*" (Mark 1:11)

I have only heard of preachers saying that because Jesus was declared as God's beloved Son before He did any ministry, therefore we are God's beloved even before we do anything. I don't think that is accurate.

Jesus lived His life fulfilling every requirement of the Law from the age of 12 (Luke 2:42). God the Father declared *"This is My Beloved Son, in whom I am well-pleased"* after Jesus fulfilled all righteousness (Mark 1:10). The Father didn't declare it because Jesus did nothing. On the contrary, the Father said it because Jesus fulfilled the Law! He was completely obedient.

Jesus pleased the Father by His works (John 8:29) so that the Father is pleased with us because of Jesus' perfect works (Ephesians 1:6). His works qualified us before the Father once and for all.

When heaven was torn open and the Spirit of God descended upon Jesus like a dove, it was a fulfillment of the prophecy by Isaiah.

*Oh, that You would **rend** the heavens! That You would come down! -* Isaiah 64:1

The word 'torn' used in Mark 1:10 is the word '**rend**' in Greek. When Jesus fulfilled all righteousness, heaven was **rent**, and God Himself (Holy Spirit) came down! From that moment onwards, Jesus walked under open heavens where healings, miracles, signs and wonders follow Him!

Something similar happened when Jesus died on the Cross.

*And behold, the veil of the temple was **torn** in two from top to bottom; and the earth shook and the rocks were split. -* Matthew 27:51

The word 'torn' here is the exact same word **'rend'** in Greek.

When Jesus died on the Cross, heaven was rent AGAIN.

Heaven was rent the first time for Jesus when He fulfilled all righteousness, and the Holy Spirit descended upon Him. Heaven was rent the second time for you and me when Jesus died on the Cross; the veil of the Temple was rent, so that the Holy Spirit could descend upon you and me. God condemned sin in the body of His Son so that the righteous requirements of the law might be fulfilled in us (Romans 8:4). The Holy Spirit is the seal of our righteousness in Christ (Ephesians 1:13-14). We are seated with Christ in the heavenly places (Ephesians 2:6). In other words, **we now walk under open heavens where healing, miracles, signs and wonders follow us!**

Jesus has qualified us to heal the sick through the Cross.

Walking Under Open Heaven

Is the Holy Spirit in you?

Then **heaven is opened for you 24/7** ------ you cannot shut it. As believers, you can't pray and fast for an open heaven. Heaven was long opened 2000 years ago when Jesus died on the Cross. It is not based on your effort or my work. It is based on Jesus' finished works on the Cross!

Stop all your religious efforts in trying to open up heavens. Stop crying *"God, rend the heavens and come down!"* He already did. He already accomplished that through Christ. What is left is mind renewal. **You need to renew your mind to see that.**

Today, we need to stop looking to healing evangelists, prophets and men and women of God, though there are things we can learn from. We need to start looking within. Jesus said, "*The kingdom of God is WITHIN you.*" (Luke 17:21). The Spirit of God has been given to you!

You don't need a minister to fly over, speak a few sessions and lay hands on you. What you need is the Minister (Christ) who died for you and paid for your healing. **Stop looking to the men of God. Start looking to the God of men!** He lives in and through you.

The body of Christ at large is still not growing in maturity because they have not learnt to know what God has already given to every single believer. This manual serves to equip believers to get their healing and to release healing to those who need it.

How To Heal The Sick?

Have you ever wondered why Jesus didn't teach His disciples how to heal the sick? You can't find it in the Bible. Jesus didn't teach, "Step One: Do this." He didn't have a five-step prayer model or something. He simply told His disciples to go and heal the sick (Matthew 10:8).

Have you ever wondered why Jesus didn't use the same method to heal the sick? There was no way His disciples could copy because He used different approaches to heal the same kind of sickness! For example, He simply said, "*Go your way...*" (Mark 10:52) and the blind man was healed. But for another blind man, He spat on the ground with His saliva and put them on his eyes (John 9:6-7).

If Jesus were to teach the methods of healing, our eyes would be fixed on the methods instead of the Man who paid for our healing. He is the Healer. If we focus on the methods, we will miss the vital element

------- our identity as sons and daughters of the Most High and our relationship with Him.

Jesus taught His disciples HOW to pray (Matthew 6:9-13) and the first two words begin with, "*Our Father*". We are sons and daughters. **Healing is in our identity. Miracles are our inheritance.** This is what we have because of who we are, and we don't change that position regardless of what we are going through. When we understand this, we will have full confidence and boldness to step out and minister healing. **Whomever we touch shall be healed!**

Let me announce to you something wonderful.

There is no method in healing.

Yes. There is absolutely no method in healing. This is good news! In other words, there is no boundary to what you can do to see someone healed. If I show you methods to heal the sick, I will be limiting your mind to these methods. Therefore, it is better NOT to teach any method, because there is really no boundary to healing.

Over the years, we have seen people healed by **words**. We have seen people healed by **laying of hand** (without saying anything). We have seen people healed by using **a tissue, a card, a mobile phone, a piece of paper, or any other object**. We have seen people healed through **video calls**, **phone calls**, **messages**, over **online customer service chatbox**, over a **distance** (without us even communicating with the person), etc. God is able to transcend every distance and barrier. **He is able to do exceeding, abundantly above all you ever ask or think, according to the power that works in you** (Ephesians 3:20).

We have seen countless healed **without us saying or doing anything**. There was a lady who received brand new kidneys through a video call. There are so many testimonies that we don't have the capacity to write them down in this manual. Testimonies are great but they are not the purpose of this manual as I mentioned in the beginning. The purpose of this manual is to teach truths and equip you.

The key to ministering healing lies in **BELIEVING**. As long as you believe, **you can do anything and the person will still be healed!**

While there is no method in healing, I would like to bring our attention to what Jesus did in the books of the Gospel.

Confronting Sickness As Though It Is A Person

If you read all the documented healings of Jesus in the Bible, you will notice that **Jesus never prayed for the sick.** To pray is to talk to God about the sickness. **Jesus always spoke directly to the sickness.** Sometimes, He simply laid His hands and the Bible doesn't record any speech. At other times, He would say words like, "*Be healed*", "*Rise up and walk*", "*Come out of him*", etc. Apostles Peter and Paul did the same thing (Acts 3:6; 14:10).

The principle comes from Mark 11:23 - "*For assuredly, I say to you, whoever says to this mountain, 'Be removed and be cast into the sea,' and does not doubt in his heart, but believes that those things he says will be done, he will have whatever he says.*"

In ministering to the sick, we do not tell God about the sickness. **We speak to the sickness directly.** Someone said, "*Don't tell God how big the mountain is. Tell the mountain how big God is.*"

Jesus commanded His disciples to "**heal the sick**" (Matthew 10:8; Luke 10:9). He didn't tell them to pray for the sick.

If your boss tells you to go and do the work, you don't go back to him and say, "*Boss, can you help me to do the work?*" He will fire you.

Similarly, God told us to go and heal the sick. We don't say, "*God, can you please heal so and so?*" **Don't ask God to do what He has already asked you to do** ----- heal the sick!

Now if you need to pray to build yourself up (Jude 20) before you minister to the sick, you can do so. In fact, on two occasions, Peter and Paul did that (Acts 9:40; 28:8) before they ministered. But when you are ministering healing, you don't pray. You confront.

We need to confront every sickness as though it is a person. This is why you speak directly to it, if you use words. If you don't use words, you need to know that the Spirit of Life that flows from you will crush the sickness.

*How God anointed Jesus of Nazareth with the Holy Spirit and with power, who went about doing good and **healing all who were oppressed by the devil**, for God was with Him.* - Acts 10:38

Jesus healed all who were oppressed. In other words, sicknesses and diseases are part of the oppression. Whoever is sick is being oppressed. And the oppressor is the devil. To put it simply... sicknesses and diseases are from the devil, whether they are caused directly or indirectly by him.

This is why when you minister to the sick, you confront the sickness as though it is the enemy. You drive him out. You get him out. If a dog bites your child, you won't be nice to the dog. You won't say, "*Excuse me, doggy... can you please let go of my child?*" No way! You will drive the dog away boldly!

Similarly, have the same attitude when you are dealing with sickness and ministering to the sick. The sick person is not your enemy. The sickness is.

"You might think by the way I went about praying for the sick that I was sometimes unloving and rough, but oh, friends, you have no idea what I see behind the sickness and the one who is afflicted. I am not dealing with the person; I am dealing with the satanic forces that are binding the afflicted". - Smith Wigglesworth, the late British faith healer (1859-1947)

Are The Manifestations Important?

A lot of the charismatics like to focus on manifestations. By the term 'manifestations', I'm not referring to the healing itself. I'm referring to visible or sensational substantiations of the healing.

While ministering to the sick, you and/or the recipient may feel one or more of the followings:
- Heat
- Tingling
- Electricity
- Wind
- Cold
- Peace

The list is not exhaustive.

You and/or the recipient may feel NOTHING at all too. That is **NOT** an indication that healing did not take place.

Years ago, I would feel heat on my left palm whenever I was in the proximity of someone who needed healing. The nearer I was to the person, the more intensified the heat would be. I enjoyed it because I could easily recognize who needed healing. After a period of time, this feeling disappeared totally.

I asked God, "*Can you give me back?*" He replied, "*That was grace. Now it's time for you to walk by faith.*"

From then on, I didn't feel anything for 90 over per percent of the healings that I ministered.

Healing is by grace through faith. It is not by sensations or the so-called 'manifestations'. Whether you and/or the recipient feels anything, it is not important. **We are called to walk by faith**, not by sight. **The fact that Jesus didn't talk about such sensations/manifestations reveals that it should NOT be the focus.**

What Are You Thinking When Ministering To The Sick?

I had tried all kinds of ways in the past while ministering to the sick, largely due to the teachings and books that I had read. I had tried to push the power through my arms as though I was an Iron Man; I tried to imagine rivers flowing through my hands; I tried to think about taking spare parts from heaven to put into the body of the sick who needed healing; I tried to raise my voice as loud as possible, etc. By the way, raising your voice doesn't get anyone healed. I think it's more for helping you get stirred up than helping the sick get healed.

Stop all these. They are not in the Bible. The Gospel is simple. Healing is simple. Don't make it complicated. If these are important, you would see Jesus and His disciples doing them. These are but man-made ideologies.

The challenge we have when we minister to the sick is our mind. If we don't take hold of our mind, it will wander. More often than not, it starts to operate from the carnal realm (see Chapter 4). The enemy will want to pull you to that realm. The next minute you'll be thinking, "*What if it doesn't work?*"

For to be carnally minded is death; but **to be spiritually minded is life and peace**. - Romans 8:6

If you stay in the carnal realm, it won't produce life and healing to the recipient. Instead, stay in the spiritual realm. The spiritual mind will produce life and peace.

When you minister to the sick, **keep your mind on Christ alone**.

You will keep him in **perfect peace**, *whose* **mind is stayed on You**, *because he trusts in You.* - Isaiah 26:3

I have realized that Galatians 2:20 helps me most when it comes to ministering healing to the sick. I'm not sharing this as a method, but a personal revelation that God has taught me some time ago. I used to think that it only applies to character. Little did I realize that it is applicable to other areas such as healing too.

I have been crucified with Christ; it is no longer I who live, but **Christ lives in me**; *and the life which I now live in the flesh* **I live by faith in the Son of God**, *who loved me and gave Himself for me.* - Galatians 2:20

When you are standing there to minister to the sick, you need to get 'you' out of the way. We can be so self-conscious that we start thinking about *"What if it doesn't..."*, *"Me... I... me..."*, *"How can I do this*?" It has nothing to with you, because you have died and you no longer live!

The more you get yourself out of the way, the more Christ can have His way. Stop thinking about you. In fact, that's how anointing flows. You don't need more anointing. Stop asking God for more. That's not biblical. God has already given you His fullness (John 3:34; Colossians 2:9-10; 1 John 2:27). You have the fullness of God's anointing.

What we need is to let the fullness of God's anointing flow out of us into the life of the recipient.

So when you are standing there to minister to the sick, you need to know that the One who has the experience of healing every sickness and disease **lives IN you**. The One who has the experience of raising the dead **lives IN you**. Christ Himself lives in you!

All you need to do is simply **believe** ------- '*I live by faith in the Son of God...*'

Note: Some say that it should be translated as '*I live by the faith of the Son of God*'. That is not true. In the Greek, 'of' and 'in' in this verse are interchangeable. We were never told in the Scriptures to live by the faith of Jesus. It is always faith **IN** Jesus (Acts 3:16; 24:24; Hebrews 11:6; John 6:29). Besides, if you are living by the faith of Jesus, you must be seeing 100% healing 100% of the time, because that's what the faith of Jesus did!

When ministering to the sick, you believe that you are standing there as Christ ministering to the sick, because Christ in you will manifest out of you to touch sick. This is identity!

And make no mistake... the Christ that was in John G Lake, is the same Christ that is in you; the Christ that is in Benny Hinn is the same Christ that is in you; the Christ that is in the healing evangelist (whomever you admire) is the same Christ that is in you! And the One that is in you is greater than the one (devil; sicknesses and diseases) that is in the world (1 John 4:4)!

Freely & Effortlessly

Heal the sick, cleanse the lepers, raise the dead, cast out demons. **Freely** *you have received,* **freely** *give.* - Matthew 10:8

The word 'freely' in Greek means 'a gift that is unearned and undeserved.' It can also mean 'effortlessly'. The context of this passage talks about healing, deliverance and raising of the dead. Not only does it talk about the position for receiving miracles, but it also talks about the position for giving miracles.

Freely.

Effortlessly.

In other words, don't try hard to get people healed. If you find yourself trying, you have already taken the position of striving. It is meant to be effortless. The way you receive salvation of your spirit is effortless ----- you just believe it. The way you 'give' healing should also be effortless. I don't plan to share many testimonies in this manual. But for the sake of this principle, I will share the following testimony.

I was at a shopping mall when I saw a young chap on the wheelchairs. I approached him and asked, "*Hey, what happened to you?*"

He answered, "*Well, I am diagnosed with multiple sclerosis and I couldn't walk for more than 10 years.*"

MS is an autoimmune disease where the insulating covers of nerve cells in the brain and spinal cord are damaged. Many of the patients cannot walk and it will only get worse because there is no cure.

I squatted and placed my hands on his knees. I said, "*Be healed.*" That's it. I didn't say more than those two words. Suddenly, his eyes were wide in amazement. He exclaimed, "*Bro! What did you do to my body? I'm feeling electricity all over my body!*"

I replied, "*God is healing you. That's healing all over you right now.*" I added, "*Get up and walk.*"

Immediately, I lifted him from the wheelchair and supported him as he took the first couple of steps. Then, he began to take another step on his own. Followed by another one... and this continued for a distance!

Overjoyed, he said, "Oh my gosh... what is happening? I can feel the strength in my knees and legs. This is impossible!"

It only took a believer to lay hands on him to be healed and set free. It was **effortless**.

Healing is effortless because every effort has been paid for at the whipping post by our beloved Savior and Lord Jesus Christ. He took the stripes, so that you and I can be free.

You Don't Need Both God's Permission and Man's Permission

God's will and permission for the sick to be healed were long established 2000 years ago when Jesus took the stripes at the whipping post. Read Chapter 2 again. Be settled once and for all. You can minister to the sick anytime, for you have been given the Great Commission (Matthew 28:18-20; Mark 16:15-18). **The Great Commission is the Great Permission to heal the sick!**

Do you need man's permission to minister healing to them?

Out of courtesy and respect, it is always good to ask before you minister healing to them. Nonetheless, you don't need their permission and approval to drive out their sickness. I have seen people healed even when they rejected my ministry to them. They said '*No*', but I still ministered from a distance and saw them healed.

Jesus delivered the demon-possessed man (Mark 5:7-8) without his permission. The man didn't ask for deliverance, but he was still delivered. The lame man outside the Temple did not ask for healing. He wanted money (Acts 3:1-10). Peter still ministered healing to him and he was healed. If the dead couldn't give any permission but were still raised from the dead (Mark 5:35-43; Luke 7:11-17; John 11:33-44), you don't need the sick to give any permission for them to be healed.

Some people may prefer to stay sick for various reasons such as sympathy, insurance payout, charity and welfare, etc. Sometimes, they do not want the healing because they are blinded by the devil (2 Corinthians 4:4). However, we have the authority in Christ to drive out sicknesses and diseases, for these are oppression from the enemy (Acts 10:38). We have the power to set the captives free.

Even if someone says '*No*' to healing, you can still minister healing and set him or her free. You don't need his permission. **The authority and power that we have in Christ are over the devil and his oppression**.

Minister Again And Stand In Faith

Sometimes, people don't receive the complete manifestation of their healing after we have ministered to them. What should we do?

It's pretty simple. **Minister again.** You don't have to change the way you do it. Just do it again.

*So He took the blind man by the hand and led him out of the town. And when He had spit on his eyes and **put His hands on him**, He asked him if he saw anything. And he looked up and said, "I see men like trees, walking." Then **He put His hands on his eyes AGAIN** and made him look up. And he was restored and saw everyone clearly.* - Mark 8:23-25 (emphasis added)

Jesus ministered to the blind man and he was partially healed. Jesus ministered **AGAIN**. He did the same thing again.

If Jesus could minister twice, I guess we can minister twice, thrice, or even many times!

Each time when you minister again, you are not doing it because it is not working. You are doing it because you believe it is ALREADY working. You are 'adding' to it.

Even if you don't see any visible improvement, do not shrink back and think, "*Man, it's not working.*" Instead, continue to stand in faith and do not move in your position of that belief.

Read the **fig tree principle again** that I shared in Chapter 3. It applies to our ministry to others too.

We have seen people completely healed when they reached home. We have received testimonies from people that they were totally healed on the next day or two. There weren't any changes when we ministered to them. But the healing happened suddenly when they left!

By His stripes, they are healed!

TODAY Is The Day

Today is the day to walk in your identity as a believer.

Today is the day for you to lay hands on the sick and see them healed.

Today is the day for you to go out into the streets and **START ministering to the first person you see who needs healing.**

It is too late to back off. You have read the manual until here. You have read the truth. You have known the truth. The Holy Spirit is convicting your heart with the truth right now, and I pray that there is no rest until you do it. You can't live in ignorance anymore. You have been given the responsibility and the truth to heal the sick as a believer of Christ. You need to step out and start.

If you don't lay hands and minister to the sick, they will surely die. They don't have a chance. But if you lay hands on them, they will live. **The possibility of them staying alive should far outweigh your fears of stepping out.**

The enemy will resist you. He doesn't want you to step out. He doesn't want you to see your first healing in the streets. He knows that once you witness the first healing, nothing can stop you. He is defeated. He is a liar. Don't listen to him.

Christ in you is the Hope of glory and Christ working through you is the manifestation of that glory. Someone out there is waiting for you to minister to him or her. You are the answer to their problem. You are the solution. God has put the kingdom within you. Go out there and manifest the kingdom of love and power! Lay hands on the sick and see them healed!

Get a buddy and do it together if it helps. Remind each other to keep going at it. We are called to set the captives free. The sick are oppressed. They are in captivity. You can set them free!

Remember: There is no hard and fast rule when it comes to healing. Whatever approach you feel led to do when you are ministering to the sick, just do it! Ultimately, it only lies with you believing that nothing is impossible in and through Christ. Every sickness and disease must flee!

WARNING

If you are still seeking healing, I strongly encourage you **NOT** to proceed to Chapter 6. Stay in Chapters 1 to 5. **Read them again. Meditate on the Scriptures. Digest and mull over them slowly.** It is not about getting more knowledge into your head or gathering more information quickly. It is about **gaining understanding in your heart**.

I will say it again -------- if you still need healing for your body, **STAY** in Chapter 1 to 5! The last chapter **may backfire** if you are not ready.

CHAPTER 6:

The Great Mystery

When it comes to healing, it is natural for us to have this burning question at the back of our mind.

"Why are some people not healed?"

"If healing is God's will and desire, why can't they be healed?"

It is always good to ask sincere questions. Especially deep questions. The disciples always asked Jesus questions when they were baffled and when they did not understand. Jesus always explained to them throughout the books of the Gospel. He never brushed them aside. Why? Questions unanswered can become a hindrance to our faith journey. They may even result in discouragement, bitterness and anger towards God, if we don't deal with questions properly.

The Word Defines Our World

"You know... so and so were not healed. In fact, they died. They had faith. They were men and women of God."

Does this sound familiar? I have heard that many times.

My responsibility is not to question what happened to these people. I'm not called to dig out the causes. I'm called to know Jesus, because He is the Answer. My responsibility is to find out what the Word of God says and stick with what it says. **If God says it, that settles it**. If God is unchanging, then His Word is unchanging, regardless of my situations or experiences.

We are not called to live by experience. **We are called to live by the Word** (Matthew 4:4).

Besides, I am not bothered by people's experiences. They can have scores of experiences, but if any of the experiences is not according to the Word, I will disregard it, no matter how 'glorious' it seems to be. Experiences must not be the teacher of truth. **The Word is the teacher of truth** (2 Timothy 3:16-17; John 1:14; 8:32; 14:6; 16:13; 17:17).

We cannot afford to allow our experiences or other people's experiences to alter the truths found in the Word of God. Instead, our **experiences must always line up with the Word**. If they have not, we need to stand firm and keep believing in the truth (John 8:32) until our experiences are aligned to it.

At the end of the day, even IF I leave this world without my experience fully aligned to the truth, it doesn't change the fact that **truth is still the truth**. My life and your life are not the ultimate examples. Jesus' life is!

Don't let what you are going through define you and become your identity. Let what Christ has gone through define you and your identity. Let the stripes and the Cross of Jesus define your position as His sons and daughters ------- healing and health are yours!

There are many books, sermons and teachings that give 1000 reasons why people don't get healed. And you can't find these excuses in the life of Jesus. Whatever that is not in the Word should not be in your world of belief. Cast them aside.

Healing Is Not A Mystery

On the other hand, there are some popular teachings that say that healing is a mystery of the kingdom of God. They claim that it is humility to acknowledge that we don't know everything. For example, when they minister to the sick and the sick is not healed, they say, "*I don't know. It's a mystery.*" They like to add, "*Well, if your puny little brain can figure God out, then you become god and He is not.*"

Some even quote from Isaiah 55:8-9.

"For My thoughts are not your thoughts, nor are your ways My ways," says the Lord. "For as the heavens are higher than the earth, so are My ways higher than your ways, and My thoughts than your thoughts."

But the verse is not talking about the mystery of God which we cannot understand. It is talking about God's perspective, which is different from men's perspective. God is saying, "*I don't think like you.*" It doesn't mean that we cannot comprehend what He thinks. We just have to set our mind on what He thinks (Colossians 3:1). An example is how God views every sickness on the same level, as what I wrote in Chapter 3.

In fact, Jesus Himself told His disciples that they had been given the mysteries of the kingdom (Matthew 13:11). However, the disciples still had things that they didn't know (John 16:12) because they didn't have the Holy Spirit. But when the Holy Spirit comes, they would know all things (John 16:13-15; John 14:26). Even apostle Paul said that we have the mind of Christ (1 Corinthians 2:16) and that we can know the deep things of God.

*But God has revealed them to us through His Spirit. For the Spirit searches **all things, yes, the deep things of God**. For what man knows the things of a man except the spirit of the man which is in him? Even so no one knows the things of God except the Spirit of God. **Now we have received**, not the spirit of the world, but **the Spirit who** *is from God, that we might know the things that have been freely given to us by God.* - 1 Corinthians 2:10-12

While it is indeed humility to acknowledge that we don't know everything and we don't have everything figured out ------ because we are still growing to know God better each day; **it is NOT humility to push aside something as mysterious if God has already shown us clearly in His Word**.

Jesus healed ALL who came to Him (Matthew 8:16-17; Acts 10:38). So did the disciples (Acts 5:16; 28:9). To say that it is a mystery when someone is not healed is to **INDIRECTLY** put the responsibility and blame back on God. He does not lie when He already said, "*By His stripes, you were healed.*"

When someone is not healed, the equation is never on God's side. Because if Jesus were to stand there to minister to that same person who is sick, he or she will be completely healed.

If the sick person is not healed, it's because he didn't have Jesus standing in front of him. He got you! Let me submit to you the reality: **the equation is on our side**.

This reality can be harsh and difficult to swallow. Most healing ministers will not want to acknowledge this. **But truth is still truth and it has to be spoken**. I rather that people get mad at me than to hide the truth and be a man-pleaser. It takes humility for one to acknowledge that he is responsible when someone whom he ministers to is not healed.

When someone I minister to doesn't get healed, I usually always apologize. I will say something like, "*I'm sorry that I didn't see you healed. If Jesus were to stand there in person to minister to you, you will be 100% healed. But instead of Jesus, you had me standing there. And I'm still growing unto Him. I'm still learning to represent Him well. Listen. God wants you healed. So please, continue to believe and continue to let other believers minister to you."*

I rather that the person and his family get mad at me than having them get mad at God. It is not God's fault! Some of these sick ones and their families are not born again. What if they get mad at God and turn away from knowing Him? That will cost them eternity!

God, by His grace, chose me to represent Him and minister to the sick. But I don't always represent Him perfectly. Sometimes, some don't get healed. That's not an accurate representation of God. Jesus healed ALL.

But I don't back off. I don't beat myself down. For I have seen way too many healed to change my mind on this. But there are still more I have yet to see. And I know that it has nothing to do with 'God's mystery'.

In fact, it is pride to brush it off as 'mystery' when it is not. **We need to humble ourselves and acknowledge that we are still growing to be like Jesus.** I count it a privilege to go back to the place of intimacy and know Him deeper, so that I can represent Him more accurately.

IMPORTANT: Do not take the burden of not seeing someone healed upon yourself after you have ministered to him or her. Do not beat yourself up. Instead, strengthen yourself even more in the Lord. Take this as an opportunity to know Him even more!

A Biblical Response To The So-Called Mystery

There was an incident recorded in the Bible where Jesus gave an answer when someone wasn't healed. It is the only record in the book of the Gospel. It can be found in Matthew 17.

*And when they had come to the multitude, a man came to Him, kneeling down to Him and saying, "Lord, have mercy on my son, for he is an epileptic and suffers severely; for he often falls into the fire and often into the water. So I brought him to Your disciples, but they could not cure him." Then Jesus answered and said, "O **faithless and perverse generation**, how long shall I be with you? How long shall I bear with you? Bring him here to Me." And Jesus rebuked the demon, and it came out of him; and the child was cured from that very hour. Then the disciples came to Jesus privately and said, "**Why could we not cast it out?**" So Jesus said to them, "**Because of your unbelief**; for assuredly, I say to you, if you have faith as a mustard seed, you will say to this mountain, 'Move from here to there,' and it will move; and nothing will be impossible for you.* - Matthew 17:14-20

The disciples had been given power and authority to cast out ALL demons and to heal ALL sicknesses and diseases (Luke 9:1; Matthew 10:1). That's just like us as believers in Christ. We have Christ's authority (Matthew 28:18-20) and power (Acts 1:8) to do the same (Matthew 10:8; Mark 16:17-18).

Yet in this incident, they couldn't cast out the demon. They couldn't heal the boy (Matthew 17:16).

Therefore, Jesus answered and said, "*Oh boy, it's a great mystery of the kingdom.*"

Did Jesus say that? By no means!

"You know what? This demon is too powerful for you."

"Oh, it must be a generational curse."

"Well, it's due to unconfessed sin!"

"Hmm... you see... it's because the boy's father did not have faith. He didn't believe."

"Beloved disciples... you guys have done your part. Well done."

"I don't really understand. I haven't gotten it figured out."

"I don't know everything."

"It's not My responsibility, you know?"

"Sometimes, healing doesn't happen. Anyway, if the boy dies, it will be Ultimate healing!"

"You know... in spite of all these.. God is still good. He is still Love. God is good... all the time..."

"You guys have prayed and ministered. Your job is done. Leave the rest to God. It's His job to heal."

Did Jesus say any of the above? **NO!**

Yet we come out with plenty of excuses when healing doesn't take place.

Look at what Jesus said in verse 17. *Then Jesus answered and said,* *"O **faithless and perverse generation**, how long shall I be with you? How long shall I bear with you? Bring him here to Me."*

Jesus wasn't rebuking the father nor the multitudes. In fact, He often moved with compassion for them (Matthew 9:36; 14:14). He knew they were helpless, like sheep without a shepherd.

Jesus was rebuking His disciples, who had the authority and power to heal the sick, but they failed to do so. His response in verse 17 was an answer for verse 16 - *"So I brought him to Your disciples, but they could not cure him."*

The word '**perverse**' in Greek is '**to distort the purpose and plans of God.**' God's will and His plan are to heal the sick. By failing to heal the boy, it was a distortion of the purpose and plans of God. Jesus was saying something like, *"You are misrepresenting the perfect will of God, which is to heal every single time."*

Jesus said, *"Bring him here to Me."* He was going to present the perfect will of God in this matter. Where the disciples couldn't, He did.

Jesus always manifested the perfect will of God because '*the Son can do nothing of Himself, but **what He sees the Father do**; for whatever He does, the Son also does in like manner.'* (John 5:19)

We sometimes don't manifest the same perfect will, because we are not always seeing what the Son sees, not because there is a mysterious way of God that we cannot comprehend. We don't have a God who plays hide-and-seek. He has made Himself known fully in the Person of Christ.

Jesus rebuked the demon (Mark 9:25). It came out of the boy and the boy was healed.

The disciples obviously wanted to know the reason why they couldn't heal the boy. I mean, these guys had great track records. This is the same burning question that most of us have.

Why is he not healed?

Why is he still sick after I have ministered?

*Then the disciples came to Jesus privately and said, "**Why could we not cast it out?**"* - Matthew 17:19

Jesus didn't give a list of reasons like we do. He didn't give that list of excuses that I mentioned earlier. We like to find excuses for the lack of power that we walk in. Jesus did NOT.

What Jesus replied is what we dislike to hear most.

*So Jesus said to them, "**Because of your unbelief**; for assuredly, I say to you, if you have faith as a mustard seed, you will say to this mountain, 'Move from here to there,' and it will move; and nothing will be impossible for you.* - Matthew 17:20

Because of your unbelief. Period.

It matches what He said earlier in verse 17 - " *O **faithless** and perverse generation..."*

Unbelief.

This answers the burning question that we all have.

"Why is he not healed?"

"Because of your unbelief."

Because you allow what you see visibly to affect you. Because you allow what you see in the sick boy to overwhelm you, instead of letting what God sees overwhelm you.

The disciples were overwhelmed by what happened to the boy, instead of being overwhelmed by the love and the power of God. They saw the problem but they failed to see what Jesus saw (John 5:19). Jesus always sees what the Father sees. When the disciples failed to manifest God's perfect will to the demon-possessed boy, Jesus came down from Mount Transfiguration (Matthew 17:1) bringing the Father's perspective. **While the disciples couldn't, Jesus manifested the perfect will of God by healing the boy and setting him free.**

Note: Jesus didn't say, "*Because of your lack of faith.*" He said, "***Because of your unbelief.***" The disciples had faith to heal the sick and cast out demons. They had good success (Luke 10:17). But they couldn't heal the boy, not because they didn't have faith, but because they had unbelief - failing to see what Christ sees.

The degree of faith is not an issue when it comes to healing. Jesus said this right after He talked about unbelief, "*...if you have faith as a mustard seed, you will say to this mountain, 'Move from here to there,' and it will move; and nothing will be impossible for you.*"

A mustard seed is extremely small. In other words, even if you have a very small degree of faith, nothing will be impossible for you. Mark 11:23 says, "*whoever says to this mountain... and **does not doubt in his heart**, but believes that those things he says will be done, he will have whatever he says.*"

It's simply about believing (Mark 5:36) **without doubting**. For doubting has to do with unbelief.

"Believe your beliefs and doubt your doubts." - F.F. Bosworth, the late American faith healer (1877-1958)

The problem does not lie with any degree of faith. It lies with doubting (unbelief). When we don't see the sick healed after ministering to them, it is because of unbelief -------- we fail to see what Christ sees!

*But let him ask in faith, **with no doubting**, for he who doubts is like a wave of sea driven and tossed by the wind. For **let not that man suppose that he will receive anything** from the Lord; he is a double-minded man, unstable in all his ways.* - James 1:6-8

*For indeed the gospel was preached to us as well as to them; but the word which they heard did not profit them, **not being mixed with faith** in those who heard it.* - Hebrews 4:2

Unbelief nullifies the Word of God.

Notice, doubting is from the heart (Mark 11:23). Unbelief is from the heart, just as believing is from the heart. In other words, your mind can say, "*I believe. I believe*", but unless your heart believes, you won't see the mountain (sickness) moves.

Mountain-moving faith is not just about what you say and what you think. It is proved by the mountain moving! If believing is present, **the mountain WILL move**. However, if the mountain doesn't move, it means there is unbelief! Your believing is not proved by you saying that you believe. **Your believing is proved by the mountain moving.** This is a hard message for many to hear. But truth has to be spoken, regardless of whether people are offended or not.

On the other hand, your mind can say, "*I don't believe. I don't think I can.*" But if the mountain (sickness) moves, it means that your heart actually believes. For our heart and our mind are not always in agreement.

IMPORTANT: The issue never lies with the sick. It lies with the one ministering ---- you and I. Never tell the sick that they don't have faith! Jesus never put any burden or responsibility on the sick. Even when the sick didn't believe (Mark 5:35-42; 9:22-24), Jesus didn't say anything about them, because He always believed (Mark 5:36; 9:23) and healed them.

Removing Unbelief

Jesus seemed to give the tool for His disciples to deal with unbelief.

So He said to them, "This kind can come out by nothing but prayer." - Mark 9:29

Some say that 'this kind' is referring to the unbelief that the disciples had. *"This kind of unbelief can come out by nothing but prayer."* However, if we read in context (Mark 9:28), Jesus was actually talking about the demon.

No. He wasn't saying that some demons require special prayer to be cast out.

He was saying something like this in full context, *"You cannot cast this demon out because of your unbelief (Matthew 17:20). So you need to pray."*

To put it simply.... *"This kind (of situation that caused you to have wrong perceiving in the mind) can come out by nothing but prayer."*

The disciples were so caught up with what they saw in this demonic situation ------ the boy was convulsing non-stop, that they failed to perceive what Christ perceived. They were moved by what happened to the boy, instead of being moved by the Father. They failed to see what Jesus saw!

Why did Jesus tell them to pray? The place of prayer is the place of communion. Jesus Himself stayed in **the place of intimacy and communion with the Father**, so that He could always see what the Father sees (John 5:19). In fact, He was in communion with the Father at Mount Transfiguration (Matthew 17:1-2) before this incident. He came down from the mountain (Matthew 17:9) bringing the Father's perspective to the boy and healed him.

Jesus was giving His disciples the tool of **prayer to deal with their unbelief**, so that they could heal the sick and cast out demons in the future, if they were ever faced with a similar incident.

When we get to the place of intimacy and communion with the Father, we learn to see what He sees (2 Corinthians 3:18). And when we see what He sees, unbelief has to go. Nothing will be impossible for us (Mark 9:23; Matthew 17:20).

And do not be conformed to this world, but **be transformed by the renewing of your mind**, *that* **you may prove** *what is that good and acceptable and perfect will of God.* - Romans 12:2

Jesus' mind was so renewed that His whole body was transformed (same Greek word as 'transfigured') in Matthew 17:2. He always **proved** the good and acceptable and perfect will of God.

We are called to follow Jesus and be like Him. Hence, we are not called to determine what the will of God is. His will is already revealed and established in His Word. **We are called to prove His perfect will**. Renewing our mind to see what Christ sees is the answer to the manifestation of His perfect will.

We need to grow in seeing what Christ sees so that we can manifest what He manifests ----- the good and acceptable and perfect will of God. The way to grow is to know and see His love for us on the Cross, because faith always works through love (Galatians 5:6).

Tearing Down Our Self-Preservation

Today, at the Christian funerals of people who died of sickness, it is not uncommon to hear pastors or brethren preach, "*God has taken our brother so-and-so back. He has finished the race and fought a good fight.*" It sounds good. It appears comforting. But that's not the truth. It's called self-preservation.

God did not take him back. He is the Giver of Life (John 10:10), not the taker. God simply received the brother back, because we failed to minister healing to him. If Jesus were there at the funeral, the funeral service would end immediately.

Apostle Paul said that he finished the race and fought a good fight (2 Timothy 4:7-8), because he had completed God's assignment for his life. He chose the time to die as a martyr (Philippians 1:21-26; 2 Timothy 4:6) after completing his race. We cannot simply apply what Paul said to every person who died of sickness. That's presumptuous!

Yes, this is a tough message. Everybody likes to say something nice and look good. Someone has to speak up and say the truth. Jesus ruined every funeral He attended. He raised them from the dead. Premature death due to sickness is never God's will. It is not God-ordained death.

Not every death is God-appointed. People love to quote Hebrews 9:27 when someone dies. The verse says that '*it is appointed for men to die once...*" But it doesn't say *WHEN* they are to die. Stop putting words into the mouth of God where He didn't say.

We need to go after the Word more than ever before. We need to be more zealous for the truth more than ever before. We cannot be satisfied with what we have right now. Jesus paid for us to walk in healing and health. We need to go after everything that Jesus has paid for, everything that He has provided by His stripes and the Cross!

Reminder: If someone is not healed when we minister to them, it is not for us to beat ourselves down. If we don't beat ourselves down for not walking in 100% unconditional love yet, neither should we condemn ourselves for not walking in 100% power yet. In reality, we are not perfect yet. But we can keep growing unto Him.

More Questions: Healing In The Missions Fields

Have you ever questioned why healing seems to take place 'more easily' in the missions fields such as third world countries and rural areas, as compared to our own first world nation?

I asked a lot of questions. And that is the privilege of being a believer. I believe that God loves questions. The disciples asked Jesus questions when they didn't understand. They asked Him when they didn't see healing. Not once did Jesus brush them off and say, "*I don't know. It's a mystery.*"

I seek God genuinely with my heart on the questions that I have. I have many questions. When we seek Him earnestly, we will find an answer (Jeremiah 33:3; Matthew 7:7-11). God, our Father, desires to give us good things (Luke 12:32; Matthew 7:11) ----- including the answers for the questions which we are seeking.

In the missions fields, I have seen miracles happened 'faster' and 'easier'. Positionally, that shouldn't be the case. Jesus paid the same price for the whole world. He took the same stripes and went to the same Cross for first world countries just as He did for third world nations. The God in the missions fields and rural areas is the same God we serve in our nation. Therefore, we ought to have the same result.

However, experientially, we don't. And I questioned why.

I was brought to the passage where Jesus met the centurion who wanted his servant to be healed.

*Now when Jesus had entered Capernaum, a centurion came to Him, pleading with Him, saying, "Lord, my servant is lying at home paralyzed, dreadfully tormented." And Jesus said to him, "**I will come and heal him.**" The centurion answered and said, "Lord, I am not worthy that You should come under my roof. **But only speak a word, and my servant will be healed.** For I also am a man under authority, having soldiers under me. And I say to this one, 'Go,' and he goes; and to another, 'Come,' and he comes; and to my servant, 'Do this,' and he does it." When Jesus heard it, He marveled, and said to those* who followed, *"Assuredly, I say to you, **I have not found such great faith, not even in Israel!** - Matthew 8:5-10*

Jesus had wanted to go to the centurion's house and heal the servant **personally**. That's Jesus' belief ------ to go and heal him in his house. Nevertheless, the centurion believed otherwise. Being a Gentile, who was not supposed to be associated with a Jew in those days, the centurion said, "*Lord, only speak a word, and my servant will be healed.*" The centurion felt unworthy for Jesus, a Jewish Rabbi, to come to his place. But he believed in the power of Jesus' words.

The centurion's belief only required Jesus to say a word right where He was, without having Him to go to his house personally.

*Then Jesus said to the centurion, "Go your way; and **as you have believed, so let it be done for you**." And his servant was healed that same hour.* - Matthew 8:13

According to the centurion's belief, not according to Jesus' belief, **it was done!**

Imagine this with me.

You intend to visit someone's house to minister healing to him. But he gives you a call and says, *"Hey, you don't have to come. Just speak a word and I will be healed."* You speak the word and he is healed. According to his belief, not your belief, it is done!

Take the imagination a little further. A lady comes up to you and requests for healing. You are going to lay hands on her but she stops you suddenly. She says, "Let me just touch your shirt and I will be healed." So she touches your shirt and she gets healed. According to her belief, not yours, it is done!

130

Does it ring a bell? The woman with the issue of blood believed that she only needed to touch Jesus' garment (Mark 5:27) to be healed. Many people touched Him but they were not healed (Mark 5:31) because they didn't have the same expectation that the woman had. According to the woman's belief, it was done. It was only after that incident that people realized they could touch His garment and be healed (Mark 6:56). Her belief opened up the possibility for the rest to believe the same.

Whose Belief? Not Always The Minister's

Bring the whole context into the missions fields and you will get the answer as to why healing seems 'easier' in the developing nations and rural areas.

Supposed that after preaching at a healing rally in the missions fields, you want to lay hands on a guy's or a lady's stomach area to minister healing. But she says, "*Pastor (they call anyone who is preaching a pastor anyway), you don't have to lay hands. Just stand where you are at the pulpit and speak a word, and I will be healed.*" And she gets healed. According to her belief, not yours, it is done!

This tells me one thing. Although a minister should always stand in faith when ministering healing to the sick, **the sick can also believe for their healing while receiving ministry**. They can have an expectation to be healed (Mark 5:34; 10:52; Matthew 8:13; 9:29; 15:28; Luke 8:48; 17:19).

Their belief can actually 'overwrite' the minister's belief (like the centurion's and Jesus' in Matthew 8:7-8). I will share more on this later.

In fact, even if the ministers have unbelief in their hearts, the sick can still be healed because the sick themselves believed! They can have the expectation that when the ministers pray or minister to them, they will be healed. And this is powerful!

Note: Anyone who is ministering healing is a minister. By right, ministers should have faith for the sick to be healed. But it's not always the case.

As ministers, we are merely the instruments (or the medium) by which the recipients place their faith in Christ. Many of them just need a human figure to put their trust in, because they can't see Jesus in person. They look at us and think that the power of God will flow through us. It's not an accurate belief but it still works. According to their belief, it shall be done (Matthew 8:13; 9:29).

Therefore, ministers should never take credit when miracles take place, especially in third world locations. Because the people in those rural areas often believe more than we (including ministers) do. **There is so much for us to learn from them ------- simple trust and simple believing!**

Disclaimer: Healing is from God. We are just the instruments to administer it. The ultimate credit and glory still belong to God Himself. It is a privilege that He chose us to partner with Him to minister healing. Having said that, it is not uncommon for ministers to get affirmation and credit when people get healed through them. I have nothing against affirmation. But I especially dislike false humility. It is false humility to say that we are not the ones (when being affirmed) but we share the healing testimonies as though we are lifting ourselves up. People who hear and read the testimonies will surely know that it is you who ministered the healing. Thus, it is completely absurd to act humble and avoid the credit when you know on the inside that you were the one who ministered the healing and shared the testimony. Why would ministers invite the sick to come to their meetings if they don't think that God is going to move through them? It is ironic. And when the sick is not healed, they shift the responsibility away as 'God's unknown mystery on healing'. We are fast to take credit but slow to take responsibility. This should not be! Nobody likes to talk about this, but someone has to speak up.

Ministers can minister to the same exact sickness in the first world and the third world but see very different results. The reason why miracles seem 'easier' in the missions fields and rural areas is this: **People in the third world have simple faith in Jesus. They understand what it means to simply believe.** They are desperate for help. They look to the ministers for help. They honor and respect the ministers greatly, believing that God's power will flow through the ministers (though it is not always true). For many of us, we have many health alternatives. We have easy access to medical doctors. They don't! Their only hope is Jesus! It is what they believe that gives them the miracles they need.

Living in a society where people conveniently pop painkillers or panadol into their bodies when they have fever or pain, it is no wonder why we see lesser miracles in our first world countries. In developing nations and rural areas, people don't go to the doctors as conveniently as we do. It requires money. If they know that Jesus is the Great Physician, they will pursue and go after Him!

Reality: I actually know of people who like to go to the missions fields (third world) for the sake of seeing more miracles!

Unfortunately, the way in which we are being brought up in our contemporary society has somehow hindered us from seeing what God sees. Almost 99% of our local people would not consider **the option of raising the dead** when their family members and loved ones die. More often than not, our eyes are set on the reality of our world instead of the reality of His world --------- the unchanging Word of truth in the Bible.

I believe that **it is possible to see the same result in every country**, because we have the same God of love and power!

More Questions: Healing In The Masses

Have you wondered why some experience healing while some do not, during a healing meeting or rally when a minister prays for all with the SAME SICKNESS to be healed?

Can you imagine Jesus ministering from the pulpit, doing mass healing in a meeting or rally but some are not healed? Can you imagine Jesus saying *"Be healed!"* and some are not healed? I cannot imagine that.

Come on! He healed them ALL (Matthew 8:16-17; 15:30; Acts 10:38, Mark 3:10; 6:56; Luke 4:40).

So why is there a difference between Jesus and the minister at the healing meeting or rally? It's because the minister is still growing to be like Jesus. He's still growing and learning to see what Christ sees, because if he sees what Christ sees, he will manifest what Christ manifests ------ every single person in the meeting or rally will be healed!

The answer as to why the result is inconsistent in mass healing is similar to that of the missions fields.

The sick can still believe for healing even if the minister has unbelief. When the minister declares "*Be healed!*" (that doesn't mean he does not have unbelief in his heart), the sick can have the expectation to be healed. Those who believe shall be healed (Matthew 8:13; 9:29; Matthew 17:20).

A renowned healing minister in the United States spoke in a large healing meeting where I attended. He called out those who needed healing and ministered from the pulpit. Not many were healed. Realizing this, he said, "*I realize that I should have first taught on word of knowledge and healing before I called you out, so that you know how to respond and receive your healing.*" He proceeded to teach how the word of knowledge and healing works hand in hand, creating an expectation from the participants to receive their healing. After that, he called out those who needed healing and ministered from the pulpit again. This time, many were healed.

The reason why it works is very simple. The minister was relying on the recipients' faith for healing to take place. He himself did not simply believe. How do I know that? If it were Jesus, He didn't have to teach in order to see healing. Because Jesus Himself always believed (Mark 5:36; 9:23).

The teaching from the American healing minister was meant to BUILD UP the expectation and faith of the participants SO THAT they could receive their healing. Because faith comes from hearing and hearing from the Word of God (Romans 10:17). When you preach the Word before you minister healing, you have already created a 'faith' expectation in the hearers to receive their healing. Every time when we preach the Gospel, healing follows (Mark 16:20; Acts 14:3).

This is why we can preach the same exact message in our own first world country and developing countries, but you see a greater percentage/result of healing in developing places (third world nations and rural areas). The hearers from the missions fields simply believe and believe simply.

Can you imagine someone approaching Jesus for healing and Jesus says, *"Please wait. Let Me first preach the Word to you, so that you can have faith to receive My healing."* You can't find Jesus saying that anywhere in the Scriptures. Today, there are still some traditional healing evangelists who do that though ------- even when they minister to an individual or a small handful of people.

Note: I have nothing against preaching the Word before ministering healing. I am simply putting into perspective why we see different results in different settings.

Jesus didn't need to preach first because He always believed (Mark 5:36; 9:23).

Healing – Only One Side Of The Equation Is Needed

When healing takes place, it doesn't necessarily mean that the minister always believes. Sometimes, he has unbelief in his heart (and he doesn't even know it), and it is the sick himself who believes and receives healing.

The minister might think that healing happened through his laying of hands or his ministry, but it didn't. It happened because the sick believed and expected to be healed. This is why the 'credit' should not always go to the 'healer' when someone gets healed.

Why? Because it only takes **one side of the equation** for healing to take place. Let me explain a little.

Apostle Paul, seeing that the crippled man had faith to be well (Acts 14:9-10), told him to stand up and he was healed. **<u>The man had faith to be healed and was healed</u>**.

Curry Blake, the successor of John G Lake, is probably the healing minister with the most effective ministry of healing and the most consistent results of healing in the world right now. He said, "*The power of God is more mechanical than you think.*" By this, he is referring to the consistency of God who changes not.

By God's grace, healing only requires a simple equation. There is no variable because God is constant and faithful to what He has said and done. The simple equation is this... **once believing is involved, healing flows.** It happens every single time. It is always the same because God is the same yesterday, today and forever.

***Believe** on the Lord Jesus Christ, and you will be **saved**... - Acts 16:31*

*If you confess with your mouth the Lord Jesus and **believe in your heart** that God has raised Him from the dead, you will be **saved**. - Romans 10:9*

The word 'saved' for both passages in the Greek is 'sozo', which means 'saved, **healed**, delivered, protected, preserved, made whole, kept safe and sound.'

It is simple. Believe in Jesus... and you will be saved. Believe... and you will be healed.

Jesus Himself said, *"Only **believe**"* (Mark 5:36) and *"all things are possible to him who **believes**"* (Mark 9:23). He said that if you **believe**, you will receive (Matthew 21:22).

The Bible only says 'believe'. It doesn't specify who should and must believe. In other words, if there are two people involved; one ministering healing and the other receiving healing, any of the two believing will result in healing flowing. This is a powerful revelation!

Check out the simple equation below.

Minister (**believe**) + sick (unbelief) -----> **healing**
Minister (unbelief) + sick (**believe**) -----> **healing**
Minister (**believe**) + sick (**believe**) -----> **healing**
Minister (unbelief) + sick (unbelief) -----> NO healing

Without believing in the equation, healing doesn't flow, just as the salvation of the spirit doesn't if believing is not involved.

Of course, God is still God. He is sovereign. In other words, He can still do whatever He wants to do (Psalm 115:3; 135:6). I believe that He can still heal even if none of the party in the equation believes. However, in general, and in most circumstances, it only takes one party in the equation to believe for healing to take place.

Note: You can believe for your own healing like what I shared in Chapter 1-4 without the need for anyone to minister to you.

The Gospel is simple. Healing is simple. ONLY **believe** and SIMPLY **believe!**

100% Healing 100% Of The Time

For in that He put all in subjection under Him, He left nothing that is not put under him. **But now we do not yet see** *all things put under Him.* **But we see Jesus**... - Hebrews 2:8-9

God has put all things including sicknesses and diseases in subjection under Jesus' feet. He is the head and we are His body (Colossians 1:18). Because we are His body, all things are also in subjection under us (Ephesians 1:22).

Nobody has seen 100% healing 100% of the time. The Bible says that '*now we do not yet see all things put under Him.*' That's our present experience. Positionally, it is done -------- all things are put under Him. Experientially, we are seeing more and more healed collectively as the Body of Christ.

Though we haven't seen perfection in healing, we have the privilege to '**see Jesus**' who is the perfection and who has shown us perfection. Thus, we must keep growing unto Him.

Growing Unto Jesus – The Perfect Representation & The Perfect Will

We need to stop coming up with excuses and theories, and make the Bible appear so complicated. We need to stop coming out with religious reasons and start looking at the Word for what it is. The only model we are to grow unto is Jesus. We need to go after all that Jesus has paid for us to walk in.

Pride is lowering the Word to your level of experience. Humility is recognizing that your level of experience hasn't matched the Word and thus, there is growth needed.

How can we grow unto Jesus?

*I have been crucified with Christ; it is no longer I who live, but **Christ lives in me**; and the life which I now live in the flesh **I live by faith in the Son of God**, who loved me and gave Himself for me.* - Galatians 2:20

The Bible says, *'It is no longer I who live, but Christ lives in me.'* What is now in you is the divine nature (2 Peter 1:4) ----- exactly as that of Christ. When you look into the mirror, you are not seeing pimples and wrinkles. You are seeing Christ in you, the Hope of glory (Colossians 1:27).

'And the life which I now live in the flesh (referring to the body), I live by faith in the Son of God.' In other words, this life is no longer about you and me. You and I are dead. Now it is about Christ. And if it is about Christ, everything you see should be Christ. If you can see what Christ sees, you will live how He lives. Who He is, is who you are. What He has, is what you have. You and I are the representation of Jesus on earth.

We like to quote Romans 12:2, but we often miss out on the previous verse. Romans 12:2 begins with the word *'And...'* (in the Greek translation). This means that it is connected to verse one and that the former verse is needed in order to produce the latter. **Before we can renew our mind to the truth, we need to first know who we are in Christ.**

*I beseech you therefore, brethren, by the mercies of God, that you **present your bodies a living sacrifice**, holy, acceptable to God, which is your reasonable service.* - Romans 12:1

A sacrifice has to be dead. If it is still living, it is not a sacrifice. In the Old Covenant, a sacrifice was only accepted before God when the blood was shed and the animal was dead.

What does it mean to present your bodies a living sacrifice?

Galatians 2:20 says that '*I have been crucified with Christ. It is no longer I who live, but Christ lives in me.*' You and I are dead in ourselves, but we are alive in Christ. The only perfect sacrifice that is holy and acceptable to God is Jesus. On the Cross, He became the ultimate sacrifice.

The reason why we can present our bodies a living sacrifice to God is that '*it is no longer I who live, but Christ (the perfect sacrifice) lives in me*' ------ that makes me a living sacrifice, holy and acceptable to God. Because of the Cross, we can present our bodies a living sacrifice, holy and acceptable to God.

If we don't understand this truth, if we don't understand who we are in Christ before God, we will always be conformed to the patterns of this world. If we don't know who we really are and our identity, we can never see what Christ sees. And we can never get our mind renewed.

And *do not be conformed to this world, but be transformed by **the renewing of your mind**, that you may **prove what is that good and acceptable and perfect will of God**.* - Romans 12:2

To the degree our mind is renewed (seeing what Christ sees), to that degree we can prove the good, acceptable and perfect will of God. If we can see what Christ sees, we will manifest what He manifests.

*But we all, with unveiled face, beholding as in a **mirror** the glory of the Lord, are being transformed into the same image from glory to glory, just as by the Spirit of the Lord. - 2 Cor 3:18*

The point of communion is not just to behold Christ alone, who is the glory of the Lord. It's also to **behold Him IN us**. Christ in you is the Hope of glory. This is why we are beholding as in a mirror. When you look in the mirror, you see YOU.

*For if anyone is a hearer of the **Word** and not a doer, he is like a man observing his natural face in a **mirror**; for he observes himself, goes away, and immediately forgets what kind of man he was. - James 1:23-24*

In communion, we must see the Word. For the Word is Christ. And the Word (Christ) is our mirror. **When we read the Word, we are reading US.** That is our true image. Whoever Christ is, we are. In communion, we grow in the revelation of who we are because of who Christ is. When we perceive who we really are, we crush the carnal mind; we crush the wrong perception, and we live by the spiritual mind -------- the mind of Christ, so that we can perceive what He perceives. **If we see what He sees, we will manifest what He manifests**.

This is the key to manifest the perfect will of God ------- seeing every sickness crushed. This proves the good, acceptable and perfect will of God. Jesus!

Growing unto Jesus as the perfect representation is not merely seeing every sickness healed. It also means we need to love like He loved. Walking in the power that Jesus walked requires us to walk in the love that He walked. While it is possible to heal the sick and live a 'double-standard' or sinful life, it is impossible to see the consistency that

Christ had for healing unless we walk in the consistency of love like He did.

All these have to do with believing. If we believe right, we will live right.

The way to grow in our believing is to know His love and His goodness. Because you can't produce faith on your own. You can't grow your faith by any effort. You can't try harder to build your faith. It is impossible. The more we see His love and His goodness, the more we will naturally respond in faith. Faith is a response from the heart.

It is knowing Him deeper in the place of intimacy and communion where our mind gets renewed and our heart believes. When you and I are fully persuaded by His love and His goodness, faith is the only response.

*And the life which I now live in the flesh, **I live by faith** in the Son of God, **who loved me and gave Himself for me**.* - Galatians 2:20

The more I know Jesus' love for me on the Cross, the more I grow in becoming like Him. You can't grow by your own effort. You can't see what He sees by your own effort. **It has to be a revelation of His love for you on the Cross**. Because faith always works through love (Galatians 5:6). We can walk in the full representation of Christ in power and love, when we are filled with the knowledge of His love.

*To know the love of Christ which passes knowledge; that you may be filled with all the **fullness of God**.* - Ephesians 3:19

This knowing is not information or head knowledge. This knowing, 'ginosko' (in Greek), is a kind of **intimate, sexual and experiential knowing that only happens in a union**. It is possible because we are in co-union with God (1 Corinthians 6:17). And this is why communion is key to know His love.

There is so much revelation of His love for us on the Cross, that it takes a lifetime to know it. If we think that we already knew His love, we have failed to comprehend the width, the height, the length and the depth of His love.

Romans 8:39 says '*nothing can separate us from the love of God that is in Christ Jesus our Lord.*' **Nothing means nothing**. Whatever our experience tells us otherwise, the Bible says '*nothing*'. It's either we live based on our experience, or we live based on the truth in the Word. If nothing can separate us from His love on the Cross, nothing can separate us from receiving healing and ministering healing to others, if we know His love and sees what He sees. **If we see what He sees, we will manifest what He manifests.**

Let's Be Committed To Growth

Together, you and I can represent Jesus more accurately day by day. Let's be committed to growing unto all that Jesus is ------ Power and Love to the dying world. **We are the encounters that the world is looking for!**

Post Script One: Challenges In Ministering To One's Own Family And Loved Ones

Over the years, I had my share of successes and failures in ministering to my own family, especially my wife and my son. Positionally, healing should be the same for them as other people whom I ministered to. God is constant and He never changes. Jesus paid the same price for my family as He paid for the whole world.

However, experientially, I find it challenging to have the same consistency and result. The closer I am to a person, the 'harder' I see the result.

They say that familiarity breeds contempt. Others quote that "*a prophet is without honor in his own hometown.*" But this has nothing to do with healing.

One of the clearest examples of this challenge is as follows.

One day, my family and I were on a trip together with my in-laws. My mother-in-law and her helper stayed in the same family room as my family. On the second day of the trip, my mother-in-law's legs became swollen, and her helper suddenly was down with a stomach issue, resulting in nausea and vomiting.

I ministered to both of them. The helper was instantly healed. The nausea left her. She stopped vomiting. Her stomach issue was also healed.

But there was no change for my mother-in-law. Her legs were as swollen as before I ministered to her. After that trip, my wife pondered and said to me, "*I know the reason. The love you have for the helper is pure and like Jesus. But not so for my mum.*"

What she said struck a chord in me.

What I am going to share in this section is extra-biblical. You can't really find it in the Bible. This entire healing manual is built on Scriptures, except for this part, which I openly declare to you that I don't have Scriptures to verify them.

Emotional Attachment

When it comes to people who are closer to us, it is natural for us to have an emotional attachment to them. We love them. We have affection for them. Sometimes, this affection overwhelms us such that we are overwhelmed by what they are going through, instead of being overwhelmed by what Christ has gone through.

Our eyes are unknowingly fixed on their sickness instead of the Author and the Finisher of our faith (Hebrews 12:1-2). Our affection for them becomes the hindrance to our ministry to them. Sometimes, it is revealed by the unrest we have in our heart, as compared to the peace we have when we minister to strangers.

The love we have when we minister to strangers is pure and like Jesus. But the love we have when we minister to our own family and loved ones is mixed with human affection, instead of pure God's compassion.

Jesus always had compassion on people. His compassion wasn't just a feeling or human affection. God's compassion is filled with passion and action. When He had compassion on the sick, He healed them and set them free.

We need to grow to that place of compassion for every single person, including our own family and loved ones.

When we minister to them, we need to separate the sickness from the person. We need to address the sickness, instead of our loved ones. We are dealing with an oppression from the enemy (Acts 10:38). We are driving it out!

It is easier said than done. But I believe that we can all grow into that position, so that we see the consistent result for our own family and loved ones. **Healing and health belong to you and your family. Jesus!**

Post Script Two: Four Biblical Approaches To Healing

According to the Bible, we see four approaches to healing. Anyone who needs healing can use one or more of the following.

1) Laying of hands on the sick (Mark 16:17-18) ----- Usually for non-believers

This is usually for non-believers who don't know how to receive healing, though believers can also receive healing in the same approach. In this approach, we get believers to lay hands and minister healing to the sick.

2) Prayer of Faith by the Elders (James 5:14-15) ------ Usually for 'younger' believers

This is usually for believers in the Church. They may have challenges to receive healing on their own. As such, it is the responsibility of the elders in the Church to minister the prayer of faith and heal them. This also means that the elders in the Church are supposed to be men and women of faith, believing for the sick for divine healing.

If you are still seeking wholeness and haven't received the full manifestation of your healing, don't give up and don't stop getting other believers to minister healing to you. Even if some great or renowned healing evangelists have ministered to you and nothing happened, it doesn't mean they have represented God accurately. As a matter of fact, they failed to walk in the power of God and they are still growing to be more like Jesus.

However, you can continue to get others to minister healing to you.

3) Holy Communion (1 Corinthians 11:24-32) ------ Usually for believers who need something tangible

This is usually for believers who need something tangible, to feel and to see, so that they can release their faith and believe for healing.

The Holy Communion is a powerful tool for divine healing. Many believers think that the Holy Communion is only symbolic ------ pointing to the death, resurrection and return of Christ. The Roman Catholics think that the elements actually change and become the literal body and blood of Christ in reality ------- transubstantiation. The mainstream Christianity (Lutherans, Anglicans and Methodists), however, believes that the Holy Communion is a sacrament where the actual presence of Christ is present.

Whichever you believe, it is more important to see what the Word says and appropriates the benefits of the Holy Communion rightly.

First of all, Jesus did not place any qualification for partaking the Lord's Supper (Holy Communion). He said, "*This do, as often as you drink it, in remembrance of Me.*" (1 Corinthians 11:25) Apostle Paul added, '*For as often as you eat this bread and drink this cup, you proclaim the Lord's death till He comes.*' (1 Corinthians 11:26)

The main purpose of the Holy Communion, therefore, is to remember and proclaim the Cross of Christ and the Hope of His return. However, in proclaiming the Cross of Christ, we can receive by grace through faith what Jesus has done with the sacrifice of His Body and Blood.

*Therefore **whoever** eats this bread or drinks this cup of the Lord in an **unworthy manner** will be guilty of the body and blood of the Lord. But*

*let a man **examine** himself, and so let him eat of the bread and drink of the cup. For he who eats and drinks in an unworthy manner eats and **drinks judgment** to himself, **not discerning the Lord's body**. For this reason **many are weak and sick among you, and many sleep**. For if we would **judge** ourselves, we would **not be judged**. But when we are **judged**, we are **chastened** by the Lord, that we may not be **condemned** with the world.* - 1 Corinthians 11:27-32

There have been weird interpretations of the Lord's Supper, resulting in fears and even abstinence from the partaking of our Lord's goodness. Some even teach that if you don't confess your sins and 'become worthy' before you partake the Lord's Supper, you will be judged, become sick and even die early.

Nothing is further from the truth!

Firstly, God has already judged all your sins on the Cross (Romans 3:23-26; 2 Corinthians 5:19; John 5:24; Colossians 1:21-22; 2:13-14; 3:13; Ephesians 4:32; Romans 8:3-4; Hebrews 9:28). Secondly, Jesus did not come to condemn the world but to save them (John 3:17). Jesus went around healing the sick (Acts 10:38; Matthew 8:16-17). There is no way God would place any sickness or death in people! We have already established who God is in **Chapter 1**.

Thirdly, the Bible does not say that you can 'become' worthy to partake the Lord's Supper by examining yourself. You have already been justified and accepted in the Beloved (Ephesians 1:6; Titus 3:4-7; 1 Peter 2:9). 1 Corinthians 11 only uses the phrase '*unworthy manner*'. In Greek, it means the same thing ------ unworthy manner.

In other words, you can partake the Holy Communion in a worthy or an unworthy manner. This is the reason why verse 28 says, '*But let a man examine himself, and so let him eat of the bread and drink of the cup.*'

Why is that so? No one can partake the Holy Communion in ignorance, because in it, the message of the Gospel is preached: **Jesus' Body was broken and His Blood was shed for us on the Cross for the remission of sins**.

So if a non-believer partakes the elements (the Body and the Blood) and does not believe in the Gospel message, he is **guilty** of rejecting Christ (1 Corinthians 11:27; Hebrews 10:26; 10:29). If a non-believer partakes the elements with understanding and believes in the message, welcome him into the kingdom of God!

The word 'examine' in 1 Corinthians 11:28 is 'dokimazo' in Greek. It means '**to approve what is good**', '**to deem worthy**' or '**to show something is acceptable**'. In the Old Covenant, the priests examined the sacrifice to approve it, to show that it is worthy and acceptable before God. In the New Covenant, we are to examine the sacrifice -------- Jesus was the perfect sacrifice. He was approved, worthy and accepted before God.

When we examine ourselves during the Lord's Supper, we are not examining to find faults. It is not about introspection. It is about Christ-consciousness. We are approved, deemed worthy and acceptable before God because of Christ's finished works. In the Greek, it says, "*...in this manner of the bread let him eat, and of the cup let him drink.*" (1 Corinthians 11:28)

When we partake the Communion, we can be thankful and joyful, knowing that we have been made worthy in Christ to partake the elements. Appreciate His Body that was broken for you. Thank Him for His Blood that removed your sins and made you righteous in His sight.

*For he who eats and drinks in an unworthy manner eats and drinks judgment to himself, **not discerning the Lord's body**.* - 1 Corinthians 11:29

The word 'judgment' in Greek is the word 'krima', which means 'results of condemnation'. The word 'discerning' in Greek is the word 'diakrino', which means 'to distinguish'. Understanding the Greek meaning is especially important for the interpretation of this passage in 1 Corinthians 11. The English translation is not accurate in the choice of words used.

When someone partakes the Communion without rightly distinguishing (understanding) the Body and the Blood of Christ, i.e. the finished works of Christ, he drinks the **results of condemnation** to himself. What exactly is this condemnation?

*For this reason **many are weak and sick among you, and many sleep**.* - 1 Corinthians 11:30

Now Paul wasn't saying this, "*If you don't partake with the proper understanding, God will judge you and you will be sick and die early.*" We have already established many times that God Himself will not judge you with sickness and death (John 5:22; 12:47). Read the beginning of this segment on Holy Communion again if you are still uncertain. Read Chapter 1 again.

Paul was simply stating the fact that the world without Christ is going through: weakness, sickness and premature death. The people in the world are still experiencing the results of condemnation: the effects of sin (1 Corinthians 11:32) because they don't know that they have been redeemed by Christ! People perish because of a lack of knowledge (Hosea 4:6). If they know and believe in Christ and His redemptive works, they will be set free.

Hence, if we partake the Lord's Supper as though we are ignorant like the unbelievers, we will simply experience what they experience ------- weakness, sickness and premature death. That is the normal life of an unbeliever.

The opposite is also true. **If we rightly distinguish the Body and the Blood of Christ, we can experience strength, health and live a long life!**

*For if we would **judge** ourselves, we would not be **judged**.* - 1 Corinthians 11:31

The first word 'judge' is the Greek word 'diakrino', which means 'to distinguish'. This is the exact same English word 'discerning' used earlier in verse 29. The second word 'judge' is the Greek word 'krino', which has to do with judgment. The verse can be read as follows.

*For if we would **distinguish** ourselves, we would not be **judged**.* - 1 Corinthians 11:31 (emphasis added)

If we distinguish ourselves rightly in Christ -------- accepted and approved before God, we would not come under judgment. In fact, as believers, we have passed from judgment (John 5:24). If a non-believer realizes the Gospel truth and distinguishes himself in Christ, he too, would not be judged. He would be saved because he believes.

*But when we are **judged**, we are **chastened** by the Lord, that we may not be **condemned** with the world.* - 1 Corinthians 11:32

The word for 'judged' is the Greek word 'krino', which has to do with judgment. As believers, God's judgment is not condemnation and death (John 5:24). It is the good judgment in Christ. God judged us righteous in Christ (2 Corinthians 5:21) with the conviction of the Holy Spirit (John 16:8; 16:10). The word 'chasten' is the Greek word 'paideuo', which means 'to train up a child so that he matures'. The word 'condemned' is the Greek word 'katakrino', which means 'condemnation'.

God wants to train us up into maturity as sons and daughters. It is vital for us to know that we have been made righteous in Christ (1 Corinthians 1:30). When we learn and understand about the word of righteousness, we grow unto maturity (Hebrews 5:13-14) and we have the ability to discern and distinguish truths accurately.

In this way, the purpose of God training (chastening) us up is to prevent us from experiencing the condemnation that the world has -------- weakness, sickness, premature death and other effects of sin.

The Holy Communion is a powerful tool that God has provided for divine healing. It is not the elements themselves that have some kind of magical powers to heal you. **It is the knowledge and understanding of the Body and the Blood of Christ that releases wholeness to you**.

When partaking the Body and the Blood, do not rush through the process. Take the time to spend in communion with God. This is why it is called Communion. Appreciate and thank Him for the Body broken for you to make you whole. Thank Him for the Blood that redeemed you from sin and sickness to walk in divine health. You can look at my sample prayer on Page 54-55 again. But remember, don't use it as a method. Method doesn't work. It's about relationship. Commune with Him relationally.

Holy Communion done wrongly will leave you sin-conscious and condemned.

Holy Communion done correctly will leave you Christ-conscious and healed.

Jesus said that if you eat His Body and drink His Blood, you will have life and not die. (John 6:50-58)

4) Law of the Spirit of Life (Romans 8:11) ------ Usually for believers who know their identity

This is for believers who know their identity and what they have been given.

But if the Spirit of Him who raised Jesus from the dead dwells in you, He who raised Christ from the dead will also **give life to your mortal bodies through His Spirit who dwells in you***.* - Romans 8:11

The presence of the divine Life within you cannot co-exist with sickness. Because of His presence, sickness must leave. The Spirit that raised Jesus from the dead is the same Spirit who lives in you. That power lives in you. It is the Spirit of Life that imparts life to your mortal body and makes you whole. By simply believing, you can let that Life flows from within to your body, crushing every sickness and disease.

This testimony from John G Lake will help you to understand better.

Back when Dr. Lake had his healing rooms up in Spokane a woman came to the healing room to be prayed for. She'd been prayed for several times, no result, nothing changed, so finally they came to him and said, "Brother Lake, this is what we're doing, and it doesn't seem to be working. We can't just get it to."

And so he said, "Well, alright, I'll pray for her; I'll deal with her." So, they took her off to the side and he sat down next to her and he started talking to her and she said, "Yeah, I know, you know if you just lay hands and I know, yeah, and I know healing... yeah, I know." She already knew all the doctrine, she knew everything. She said, "Yeah. Everybody else has laid hands on me so just go ahead."

And he said he stopped there for a moment and said, "You're a Christian?" She said, "Well, of course I am, sure I am." Then he said, "Well you have the Spirit of God in you?" She said, "Well, of course I do." He said, "Alright, I'm not going to pray for you. I'm not going to lay my hands on you. Here's what you're going to do. I want you to go over and sit in this chair. Are you saved?"

And she said, "I've told you I'm saved." And he said, "So, Jesus lives in your Spirit?" And she said, "Yes." He said, "I want you to sit for a few minutes. I don't want you to do anything else. I'm not going to pray for you, and I don't want you to pray. I want you to just sit there and realize that as much as Jesus is in your Spirit. He wants to be in your soul and your flesh. And I want you to let Him out of your Spirit, into your flesh."

And she thought, "That's the most ridiculous thing I've ever heard."

But she sat there for a few minutes and started thinking about it. And he said, "Is Jesus in your flesh yet." And she said, "I don't understand what you're talking about." He waited a few moments. He said, "Just recognize, Jesus is in your Spirit. He wants out. Let Him out; just let Him into your flesh."

A few more minutes, he said, "So where is Jesus? Have you let Him out yet?" and this woman looked at him and said, "He is in my flesh just like He is in my Spirit." And he said, "Yeah." She said, "No He's in my flesh. Just like He's in my Spirit." And she started getting more and more excited and started saying, "I've got it. I've got it; I understand He's in my Spirit and He's in my flesh!"

And he looked at her and he said, "Well, if He is in your Spirit then death can't be in your Spirit." She said, "Well, of course not!" Lake said, "Well then, if He is in your flesh then death can't be in your flesh." She said, "That's right!" He said, "If death's not in your flesh then you can't get sick; you can't be sick." She said, "You're right. He's in my flesh and I'm healed."

She got up, healed.

Why? He didn't lay hands on her, she just recognized and let the Spirit that was in her spirit into her flesh. Now, do you realize what that means? That means that the Spirit of God in her the whole time was there to heal. The whole time.

Lake showed her a way to get healed internally, that is when she was able to release the Spirit of God out of her Spirit and let the Spirit into her flesh. - John G Lake, on Divine Healing

----

You and I can let the Spirit of God out of our Spirit into our flesh. Quit containing Him and just let Him have free course in your flesh. You will be made whole!

Post Script Three: Baptism Of The Holy Spirit

The baptism of the Holy Spirit is an area where the enemy strongly comes against. In fact, healing and baptism of the Holy Spirit are the most argued topics among the Body of Christ. We must know that our fight is not against flesh and blood, but the enemy (Ephesians 6:12). People are not our enemy. The devil is. He is trying his best to tear and divide the Body of Christ.

The reason why the enemy comes against these two topics is that they are vital to advance the Gospel of the Kingdom (Romans 15:19; 1 Corinthians 2:4-5; 4:20; 1 Thessalonians 1:5). The full message of the Gospel of the Kingdom must also include healing and power. More than 50% of Jesus' ministry throughout the books of the Gospel was on healing. Healing is thus, central to the Gospel message. No wonder the devil comes against it.

When Jesus taught His disciples and gave the Great Commission to them, He also talked about the importance of the baptism of the Holy Spirit, because in it lies the power of God.

*But you shall **receive power when the Holy Spirit has come upon you**; and you shall **be witnesses to Me** in Jerusalem, and in all Judea and Samaria, and to the end of the earth.* - Acts 1:8

The word 'power' in Greek is the word 'dunamis', which means 'power through God's ability'. It is this power that works miracles and healings (Matthew 7:22; 11:20-21; Mark 5:30; Luke 1:35).

This power is given to us as believers so that we can be effective witnesses for Jesus. In other words, the power of God will always be most evident when we are out there in the world as His witnesses (Mark 16:20; Acts 14:3).

This power is not exclusive for some. It is for ALL believers (Mark 16:16-18; see Chapter 5). It is not only a good thing. It is essential and freely given to every believer.

Before the disciples went out to fulfill the Great Commission (Matthew 28:19-20; Mark 16:15-18; Luke 24:46-47; John 20:21-23) and preach the Gospel of the Kingdom with the confirmation of signs and wonders (Mark 16:20 Acts 14:3), Jesus told them to wait at Jerusalem for the Promise of the Father.

*Behold, I send the **Promise** of My Father upon you; but tarry in the city of Jerusalem until **you are endued with power from on high.** - Luke 24:49*

This promise was spoken by Jesus earlier in John 7.

*"He who believes in Me, as the Scripture has said, out of his heart will flow rivers of living water." But this He spoke **concerning the Spirit**, whom those believing in Him would receive; for the **Holy Spirit was not yet given, because Jesus was not yet glorified**. - John 7:38-39*

This living water is different from what Jesus said in John 4:13-14. The one in John 4 is the fountain of water within a believer ------ that results in eternal life. The one in John 7 is an overflow of living water ------ that results in power.

The one in John 4 is what the disciples received when Jesus breathed into them after His resurrection.

*And when He had said this, He breathed on them, and said to them, "**Receive the Holy Spirit**." - John 20:22*

That is the indwelling of the Holy Spirit in every believer when he or she believes in Christ.

The one in John 7 is what the disciples received when Jesus was glorified (Acts 1:5; 1:8).

*When the Day of Pentecost had fully come, they were all with one accord in one place. And suddenly there came a sound from heaven, as of a rushing mighty wind, and it filled the whole house where they were sitting. Then there appeared to them divided tongues, as of fire, and one sat upon each of them. And they were all **filled with the Holy Spirit and began to speak with other tongues, as the Spirit gave them utterance**. - Acts 2:1-4*

This is the baptism of the Holy Spirit, which is different from the indwelling of the Holy Spirit. The word 'filled' in Greek is 'pimplemi', which means 'fill to the maximum'. It is used whenever it has to do with the baptism of the Holy Spirit (Acts 4:31; 9:17). When you are baptized in the Holy Spirit, you are filled to the maximum. You cannot have more of the Holy Spirit, because He comes in fullness (John 3:34) and He doesn't leak or leave you (1 John 2:20; 2:27). He has come to abide in you.

Someone used this analogy: The indwelling of the Holy Spirit is like you pouring water into a cup and filling it. The baptism of the Holy Spirit is like you putting the whole cup fully into a river of water. In fact, the word 'baptism' simply means 'immersed' or 'dip under'.

Apart from Acts 2, there were other instances on the baptism of the Holy Spirit. Read Acts 4:31; 8:14-19; 9:17-18; 10:44-46; 11:15-17; 19:1-7. It is so important that it was the first thing that the apostle Paul asked when he met some disciples (Acts 19:2).

The baptism of the Holy Spirit on the Day of Pentecost was also the fulfillment of prophet Joel's prophecy.

*And it shall come to pass afterward that **I will pour out My Spirit on all flesh**; your sons and your daughters shall prophesy, your old men shall dream dreams, your young men shall see visions. And also on My menservants and on My maidservants **I will pour out My Spirit in those days**.* - Joel 2:28-29

Apostle Peter himself said that it was the fulfillment (Acts 2:16-21; 2:38-39) of Joel's prophecy.

*But this is what was **spoken by the prophet Joel**: "And it shall come to pass **in the last days**, says God, that **I will pour out of My Spirit on all flesh.**"* - Acts 2:16-17

Today, we no longer pray for God to pour out His Spirit. **He already did on the Day of Pentecost**. The Day of Pentecost was the confirmation that we are all now living in the last days (Acts 2:17; Hebrews 1:2). Stop praying for God to pour out His Spirit. He already did 2000 years ago on the Day of Pentecost. **Now it is up to us to believe and receive it**.

How Do We Receive The Baptism Of The Holy Spirit?

Since the baptism of the Holy Spirit is a gift from God (Acts 2:38), it should be received the same way we receive salvation of the spirit and healing. It is **by grace through faith.** You cannot earn it. You cannot do anything to get it. Simply believe and receive.

In the Bible, there are two approaches to receive: either **by receiving from God directly** (Acts 2:1-4; 4:31; 10:44-46) or **by someone laying hands on you** (Acts 8:14-19; 9:17-18; 19:1-7).

You can ask God directly. He is a good Father. When you ask, He will surely give (Luke 11:11-13; 12:32). You simply receive by believing.

*And they were all filled with the Holy Spirit and **began to speak with other tongues, as the Spirit gave them utterance**. - Acts 2:4*

One of the signs of the baptism of the Holy Spirit is speaking in tongues. There are many benefits of tongues but that's not the purpose of this manual. We are not going to talk about the various types of tongues in the Bible. In this manual, we will only focus on tongues as a prayer language from the baptism of the Holy Spirit.

Apart from Acts 2:4, other instances also recorded the sign of tongues from the baptism of the Holy Spirit. Read Acts 8:14-19. Simon the sorcerer saw something manifested (Acts 8:18) from the baptism of the Holy Spirit. The Bible does not record what the manifestation was. It could either be tongues or prophecies (Acts 19:6), as these are tangible and visible manifestations.

Read Acts 9:17-18 and compare with 1 Corinthians 14:18. Apostle Paul spoke in tongues too.

Read Acts 10:44-46. The Gentiles believed and spoke in tongues. This passage also reveals that someone can receive the baptism of the Holy Spirit the moment he or she believes in Jesus.

Read Acts 19:1-7. They spoke in tongues and prophesied.

I am not here to debate whether you must have tongues or not. The main purpose of the baptism of the Holy Spirit is for power (Luke 24:49; Acts 1:8).

Having said that, as you ask God for the baptism of the Holy Spirit, you can also ask Him for tongues. He will give you and not withhold from you (Romans 8:32; Luke 12:32).

One simple approach is simply to worship Him with songs from your heart (Ephesians 5:19). After you have asked Him for the baptism of the Holy Spirit and tongues, open your mouth and worship Him from your heart. Stop singing in English. Stop singing in any language you know. Simply open your mouth and sing. Let what is in your heart come out of your mouth. Let it bubble out. Don't worry about what may come out. The Holy Spirit will give you the utterance. He is not going to control your mouth. So you have to be the one to step out in faith and act upon it. Open your mouth and sing or speak (not in English or any known language). It may come out as only one syllabus or it may be more. It doesn't matter. Just keep going. Keep singing. Keep speaking. Don't stop.

The enemy may put thoughts into your mind, *"This is fake. You are making up the words. This is gibberish. Stop it."* Do not succumb to his lies. They are subtle and they sound like you.

Do not stop. Keep stepping out in faith. As you keep going, more syllabuses or words of the heavenly language will flow out of your mouth.

What I am sharing next is extra-biblical. I don't really have the Scriptures to prove it. But it may help you.

If you are really praying in tongues, your mind should be free (1 Corinthians 14:14). Apostle Paul said that when you are praying in tongues, your spirit is praying but your mind is unfruitful. The word 'unfruitful' means 'contributing nothing'. In other words, your mind is free to think about other things, **including reading an article or a book**. So when you are really praying in tongues, you can still be reading an article or a book. Because if you are just trying to make up some words or syllabuses, your mind will be engaged and you can't focus on reading other stuff.

In a nutshell, the baptism of the Holy Spirit is freely given to every believer, so that you and I can walk in power and represent Jesus effectively as His witnesses (Acts 1:8). Believe and receive!

Baptism Of Fire?

The charismatics love to talk about the baptism of fire. They believe that it is different from the baptism of the Holy Spirit. They think that baptism of fire will give you 'extra' anointing, power and love. They would lay hands on you and say, "*Fire! Fire! Fire!*" They preach, "*You got to be baptized in fire! You will see an increase. There will be a tremendous breakthrough after today! Fire! Fire! Fire!*"

The baptism of fire is taught by them to be separated from the baptism of the Holy Spirit. It is believed that a believer needs three baptisms. Water baptism, baptism of the Holy Spirit and baptism of fire. Well, you cannot find that in the Bible.

Many of them quote from the passage in Matthew 3.

*I indeed baptize you with water unto repentance, but He who is coming after me is mightier than I, whose sandals I am not worthy to carry. He will baptize you with the Holy Spirit and **FIRE**.* - Matthew 3:11 (emphasis added)

Firstly, we have already established the truth that you cannot have an extra anointing. You already have the fullness of God's anointing, who is the Holy Spirit (1 John 2:20; 2:17; John 14:26; see Chapter 2 again).

Secondly, we need to interpret the Scriptures in context. A text without the context becomes the pretext for a proof text. Let's look at the preceding and following verses and you will get the answer.

*But when he saw many of the Pharisees and Sadducees coming to his baptism, he said to them, "Brood of vipers! Who warned you to flee from the wrath to come? Therefore bear fruits worthy of repentance, and do not think to say to yourselves, 'We have Abraham as our father.' For I say to you that God is able to raise up children to Abraham from these stones. And even now the ax is laid to the root of the trees. Therefore every tree which does not bear good fruit is cut down and **THROWN INTO THE FIRE**. I indeed baptize you with water unto repentance, but He who is coming after me is mightier than I, whose sandals I am not worthy to carry. He will baptize you with the Holy Spirit and **FIRE**. His winnowing fan is in His hand, and He will thoroughly clean out His threshing floor, and **GATHER HIS WHEAT INTO THE BARN**; BUT He will **BURN UP THE CHAFF** with unquenchable FIRE."* - Matthew 3:7-12 (emphasis added)

The context of this passage is John the Baptist preaching the baptism of repentance. Unfortunately, the Pharisees and the Sadducees didn't want to repent. John said, "*Every tree which does not bear good fruit is* *cut down and **thrown into the fire**.*" A good tree bears good fruit. A bad tree bears bad fruit. It has to do with believing. If you believe wrongly (not in Christ), you will bear bad fruit. John was referring to the Pharisees who refused to repent.

He added, "*I baptize with water unto repentance, but Jesus is coming to baptize with the Holy Spirit and fire.*" He further explained what the fire meant. Jesus would gather His people (wheat) into the barn but **burn up unrepentant ones (the chaff) with FIRE**.

The Amplified Bible says in Matthew 3:11, "*He will baptize you [who truly repent] with the Holy Spirit and **[you who remain unrepentant] with fire (judgment)**.*"

Dr. Luke recorded the words of Jesus given to His disciples in Acts 1:4-5, "*You have heard from Me; for John truly baptized with water, but you shall be baptized with the Holy Spirit not many days from now.*" Read also Acts 11:15-16.

Notice, Jesus didn't say to His disciples, "*You will be baptized with the Holy Spirit **and fire**.*" Luke omitted the word 'fire' when he recounted the words of Jesus (Acts 1:4-5; 11:15-16). Why is that so? Because **baptism of fire is reserved for the unrepentant ones**. Read the whole book of Acts and the entire epistles and you won't find a single record of any believer being baptized in fire.

The charismatics are correct in that there are three baptisms: Water Baptism, Baptism of the Holy Spirit and Baptism of Fire. But I would prefer not to be baptized in fire. Because it's the fire of judgment for the unrepentant ones. If you want the baptism of fire, go ahead. I am satisfied with the baptism of water and the Holy Spirit. Let's stay with the Bible and stop following extra-biblical stuff.

Be Filled Again And Again?

One of the questions that some believers ask is this, *"Do I need to be filled again? Do I need to receive the baptism of the Holy Spirit again?"*

A common verse that is often quoted is as follows.

*And do not be drunk with wine, in which is dissipation; but **be filled with the Spirit**... -* Ephesians 5:18

We were taught that we need to be filled with the Holy Spirit over and over again. Some even say that the Holy Spirit can leak in our lives. Therefore, we need to be filled again.

But this contradicts what Jesus said in John 3:34 where God does not give the Spirit by measure. The Holy Spirit comes in fullness. He has come to abide forever (Colossians 2:9-10; John 14:16; 1 John 2:20; 2:27). The Holy Spirit doesn't leak.

Yet some charismatic circles tell us to receive the baptism of the Holy Spirit over and over again. They don't use the word 'baptism of the Holy Spirit' to be exact. They say, "*Get filled again. Come and receive again. Come and be prayed for again. Ask God to touch you and fill you with more of Him again.*" They specifically use Ephesians 5:18 to prove that point.

Another verse that is commonly used to justify this type of 'more filling of the Spirit' is Acts 4:31. They say something like, "*The disciples were already filled in the Spirit in Acts 2:4. But now they are filled again, you know?*"

Well, you cannot build a doctrine based on what is implicit. In Acts 2:4, only about 120 disciples received the baptism of the Holy Spirit (Acts

1:15). By the time we reach Acts 4, there were already new believers being added.

*And they laid hands on them, and **put them in custody** until the next day, for it was already evening. However, many of those who heard the word believed; and the **number of the men came to be about five thousand.*** - Acts 4:3-4

New believers were added and the total number became about 5000. But Peter and John were arrested before that (Acts 4:1-3). They probably had not had a chance to lay hands on the new believers to be baptized in the Holy Spirit.

Could it be that in Acts 4:31, it was the rest of the believers receiving the baptism of the Holy Spirit?

And when they had prayed, the place where they were assembled together was shaken; and they were all filled with the Holy Spirit, and they spoke the word of God with boldness. - Acts 4:31

In fact, the Greek word used for 'filled' in Acts 2:4 and Acts 4:31 is different from the Greek word used in Ephesians 5:18. Each time when it talks about the baptism of the Holy Spirit in Acts, the word used for 'filled' is 'pimplemi', which means 'fill to the maximum'. Even apostle Paul's own baptism of the Holy Spirit (Acts 9:17) uses the word 'pimplemi.'

But in Ephesians 5:18, the word used for 'filled' is 'pleroo', which means 'to fill, to diffuse through one's soul: with everything which God wills.'

Apostle Paul wrote clearly that there is fruit produced for Ephesians 5:18. Yet the majority of the time, there is no fruit produced after people get 'spiritual high' or 'filled by the Spirit over and over again' according to the charismatic type of interpretation. People keep getting touched without transformation.

Nowhere in the epistles did Paul talk about this type of 'filling of the Holy Spirit' for the bearing of fruit, except in Ephesians 5:18. Hence, it is important to know what Ephesians 5:18 means.

Paul talked about the fruit of 'be filled with the Spirit' after Ephesians 5:18.

...speaking to one another in psalms and hymns and spiritual songs, singing and making melody in your heart to the Lord, giving thanks always for all things to God the Father in the name of our Lord Jesus Christ, submitting to one another in the fear of God. - Ephesians 5:19-21

This speaks of a transformed life. The same writer wrote in Romans 12:2 that transformation depends on mind renewal to the truth. It is in line with what Jesus said in John 8:31-32, "*If you abide in My word, you are My disciples indeed. And you shall know the truth, and the truth shall make you free.*"

I believe that what Paul really meant in Ephesians 5:18 is not, "*get touched and filled by the Holy Spirit again and again and again.*" Why is that so? Because there are already many explicit passages that show that we have already received the fullness of the Spirit. I have shared throughout the manual on that. In fact, as believers in Christ, we should never thirst again (John 4:14; 6:35; 7:37-38; Matthew 5:6 is for those who haven't received Jesus as their righteousness). Of course, we should not be satisfied with our walk with God. We need to go after everything that Jesus has paid for us to walk in.

What then could apostle Paul be referring to in Ephesians 5:18?

Ephesians Chapter 4 & 5 are Paul's instructions on walking out the Christian life. They are very practical. Paul already spoke of what Christ did for us and what we have in Christ in Chapter 1 to 3. Now in Chapter 5, he talked about living out the Christian life. The word '*be filled*' is an active, instead of a passive thing. It is similar to 'be holy' (1 Peter 1:16), 'be perfect' (Matthew 5:48), etc. In other words, it is something like "*because you are filled with the fullness of the Holy Spirit, now be filled... walk in that fullness.*"

The Living Bible translates Ephesians 5:18 as, "*be filled instead with the Holy Spirit and controlled by Him.*" In other words, "*be yielded to the Holy Spirit.*" This is similar to Galatians 5:16 where Paul said, "***Walk in the Spirit****, and you shall not fulfill the lust of the flesh.*"

What is the lust of the flesh? Paul continued in the passage below.

*Now the works of the flesh are evident, which are: adultery, fornication, uncleanness, lewdness, idolatry, sorcery, hatred, contentions, jealousies, outbursts of wrath, selfish ambitions, dissensions, heresies, envy, murders, **DRUNKENNESS**...* - Galatians 5:19-21 (emphasis added)

Compare Galatians 5:16-21 with Ephesians 5:18. We let Scriptures interpret Scriptures.

*And do not **BE DRUNK** with wine, in which is dissipation; but **BE FILLED** with the Spirit...* - Ephesians 5:18 (emphasis added)

By comparing the two passages, Paul was saying something like, "*Do not walk in the works of the flesh (which includes 'do not be drunk with*

wine'), *but walk in the Spirit (be filled or be yielded to the Spirit)* -------
for it produces fruit!"

Last but not least, the same writer, Paul said the following in
Colossians 3.

*Let the **WORD OF CHRIST DWELL IN YOU** richly in all wisdom,
teaching and admonishing one another in psalms and hymns and
spiritual songs, singing with grace in your hearts to the Lord. And
whatever you do in word or deed, do all in the name of the Lord Jesus,
giving thanks to God the Father through Him. - Colossians 3:16-17*
(emphasis added)

Scriptures interpret Scriptures.

*And do not be drunk with wine, in which is dissipation; but **BE FILLED
WITH THE SPIRIT**, speaking to one another in psalms and hymns and
spiritual songs, singing and making melody in your heart to the Lord,
giving thanks always for all things to God the Father in the name of our
Lord Jesus Christ, submitting to one another in the fear of God. -*
Ephesians 5:18-21 (emphasis added)

We can safely say that the phrase *'Be filled with the Spirit'* is the same
as *'Let the Word of Christ dwell in you.'*

To put it simply, Ephesians 5:18 is talking about *'be yielded to the
Spirit'* (which is also the Word), *'walk in the fullness of the Spirit'*, *'abide
in the Word.'* It has nothing to do with "*Come and get filled and
touched by the Spirit again and again and again.*"

Knowing our identity is important. Knowing what we have already received is vital. It's about renewing our mind to that truth. So now, we don't keep asking for more of the filling of the Spirit. Because God has already poured out the fullness of the Spirit into us. You already have the fullness. You already have been filled to the maximum. You have all the anointing that Christ has. It's not about having more. You can't. It's about surrendering more. **Now we need to yield ourselves more to Him. It's about letting Christ live in and through us** (Galatians 2:20). That is what bears fruit that lasts.

Printed in Great
Britain
by Amazon

31099134R00102